LOSE
WEIGHT.
FEEL
GREAT.
GET IN
SHAPE.

A SiMPLE GUIDE FOR WOMEN WHO ARE BUSY WITH KIDS, WORK & LIFE

MICHAEL BRIGO

R^ethink

First published in Great Britain in 2021 by Rethink Press
(www.rethinkpress.com)

Contents

Foreword

I t's no secret that women around the world are more stressed, overworked and time-poor than previous generations as they attempt to navigate the unachievable expectations of modern motherhood. Between working and balancing the needs of dependent children and the increasing health needs of their aging parents, women feel overwhelmed and neglected, with little time for themselves. It's exhausting.

Recent research by Marketing to Mums revealed that 63% of mothers feel that society does not do a good job at understanding and supporting mothers. Women have made it clear that they feel misunderstood, misrepresented and undervalued. The ongoing daily stressors and lack of support see many women in their child rearing days put everyone else's needs in front of their own. They feel exhausted and their health can be compromised. It's not surprising that many women experience difficulty in getting (and keeping) in shape and losing weight. You might be one such woman.

Is it time for change?

This book provides an opportunity to learn how to take back control of your health and deliver the greater confidence and energy you desire. Michael highlights the reasons that your previous attempts to regain your energy may not have been as successful as you would have liked. More importantly, Michael shares his five pillars to sustained success.

With so much written about weight loss and healthy lifestyles, you might be asking yourself, 'What makes this book any different?' In my view, it's the simplicity of Michael's twelve-week transformation plan. Rather than focusing on the result you might be aiming for, Michael's process focuses on small behavioural changes which amass to significant results. Throughout this book, Michael demonstrates his deep understanding of the lifestyle pressures facing women as they enter motherhood and progress through menopause.

Michael is so passionate about transforming the lives of overwhelmed women as he guides them to take back control of their health and wellbeing. It's clear he is on a mission to deliver women more confidence, strength, vitality and joy. The numerous stories of women he has worked with and the impact this work has had on these women's lives are testament to this. Their transformations are profound and go well beyond weight loss and into every area of their lives. They will inspire and encourage you as you start your own transformation. They let you know that you are not alone.

Whether you are a woman entering motherhood or a woman entering her mid-life and going through menopause, this book can change your life.

Katrina McCarter
Global motherhood expert, author, speaker
and founder of Marketing to Mums
(www.marketingtomums.com.au)

Introduction

Losing weight and getting in shape are only our goals; our *reason* for wanting these things is to feel good, both inside and out, and we're about to embark on a personal journey to achieve that.

We all have our own definition of what it means to feel good. If you are pleased with your reflection in a mirror and feel confident within yourself, you feel good inside. If you're stronger, fitter and have energy to do the things you want and you trust your body's physical condition to function well in this world, you feel good inside. Good mental, emotional and spiritual health helps you experience and express happiness, compassion, joy and love, and means you feel good inside.

If your personal definition of feeling good includes improving the health of both your mind and your body, this book will take you on a personal health and fitness journey to achieve that.

Before we begin, I would like to shed some light on who this book is for and what you can expect in the upcoming chapters. I'm a body transformation coach for women with busy lives. As a teenager I was over-weight and unhappy. I held a smile on my face to keep up appearances, but I didn't feel good about myself.

I decided to make a change – and that's where my fitness journey began.

Exercise, food, healthy habits and improving my well-being became my primary focus. I took it all on board and, with many successes and failures along the way, I finally reached my goal of feeling good about myself. I was slimmer, fitter and stronger. More importantly, I was happier, and this improved my physical, mental and social wellbeing. This transformational journey had an empowering and positive impact on me and inspired me to help others achieve their health and fitness goals.

Brigo Personal Training (BrigoPT) was established in 2015 with the purpose of improving the lives of women so they can look and feel great at any stage in life. BrigoPT works with full-time mothers, business owners, executives and CEOs who have busy lives and want to focus on their wellbeing.

An online survey of nearly 10,000 women by You-Beauty.com revealed that over 85% of the participants were unhappy with their weight.[1] Through consultations, working with clients and connecting with women, I began to see that it was harder for mothers – whether they were full-time mums, or in a profession, or both – to achieve their fitness goals than it was for many others.

Mothers expressed frustration stemming from their busy lives as they raised their children, assisted with the upkeep of their homes, ran businesses or worked in full-time jobs, and served as caregivers to their aging parents. The various challenges presented through the different stages of motherhood and life result in mothers generally having little time for themselves and consequently feeling emotionally, physically and mentally tired. This makes it difficult to find the motivation to start a fitness routine on their own. When I discovered this was a common problem it prompted me to work exclusively with mothers, so they can look and feel great at any stage in life. This, in turn, brings confidence, strength, vitality and joy.

1   V Swami et al, 'Associations between women's body image and happiness: Results of the YouBeauty.com Body Image Survey (YBIS)', *Journal of Happiness Studies* (2014), https://link.springer.com/article/10.1007%2Fs10902-014-9530-7, accessed 30 March 2021

There are three key stages in a woman's adult life, the first two experienced by women who become mothers and the third by all women. These are pregnancy (pre-/postnatal); family life, when the woman is raising children; and menopause. During these stages many women experience what I identify as the 3Cs: Change, Challenge and Comeback. They begin with various physical, mental and emotional changes, followed by the challenges that many can experience as a result of those changes and other factors in achieving their health and fitness goals. Finally, there's the comeback, when the goal is to return to some sort of normalcy in looking and feeling better and despite the struggles, powering through to get healthier, fitter, stronger and feeling good about oneself. So, what are these challenges and why is it harder for women with children to achieve their fitness goals?

I analysed comments from over 500 consultations with women aged between thirty and sixty, of whom 95% were mothers (80% working in a profession and 20% being full-time mums). The data showed that during the first stage (pre-/postnatal) on average, women put on 9.5 kg post-birth and were unable to lose that weight for an average of three years. Those with two or more children took longer to lose the weight.

Women generally seem to play a bigger role in and take greater responsibility for the care of their children. One study showed that during the second life stage (raising children), women spent 13.7 hours per week caring for their children, compared to 7.2 hours for men. The same study showed the weekly hours spent doing household chores for married mothers was 18.3 hours, while their husbands spent 9.5 hours.[2] This indicates that women are taking on a disproportionate responsibility for household chores and childcare compared to their male partners. For those who have more than one child or are single parents, that workload increases.

Why is this relevant? Women are generally the pillars of the family home and the glue that holds everything together. They often put others before themselves, especially family, leaving little time for themselves. This makes it harder for them to achieve their health and fitness goals to look and feel better.

A study showed that the average weight gain during the third life stage (menopause) is about 2–4.5 kg; however, 20% of the participants gained 4.5 kg or more.[3] Not all women experience weight gain at this time, but many do experience a change in their body shape, and for some, this change may feel distressing. The symptoms of menopause can be disruptive and get in the way of a woman's wellbeing goals. Some symptoms appear in the perimenopausal stage and

---

2   S Bianchi et al, 'Housework: Who did, does or will do it, and how much does it matter?', *Social Forces*, 91/1 (2012), pp55–63

3   R Wing et al, 'Weight gain at the time of menopause', *JAMA Internal Medicine*, 151/1 (1991), https://jamanetwork.com/journals/jamainternalmedicine/article-abstract/614449, accessed 30 March 2021

can continue for years. This can affect energy, mood, weight and other factors which can be detrimental to mental health. In addition, for those women who choose to bear children later in life, getting in shape becomes more difficult with age. Add to this the growing commitments and responsibilities that come with age and starting a fitness routine that is too complicated or difficult can become an instant barrier to doing anything at all.

This is why BrigoPT's twelve-week transformation plan was created with one theme in mind: simplicity. The plan encompasses five steps called the 5Ms: Mindset, Motivation, Meals, Move and Maximise – each are applicable to all three stages of life and will be explained in detail throughout the course of the book. The plan is designed to realistically fit into your lifestyle no matter how busy you currently are, by incorporating the 5Ms at whatever stage you're in now, whether you do it on your own or with professional guidance along the way. The 5Ms are mutually interdependent, with the purpose of allowing any woman to look great, feel good about herself and live with incredible joy.

Get ready to start your journey to looking and feeling great.

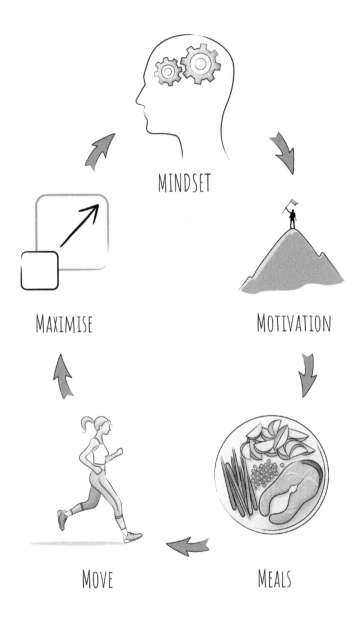

MINDSET

MOTIVATION

MEALS

MOVE

MAXIMISE

1
Mindset

The first step in the 5Ms is Mindset. Before we can dive into the nitty gritty of exercise, nutrition, top tips, and dos and don'ts, let's go right to the genesis of it all and explore why this is important.

To achieve your goals, you're going to make improvements in your lifestyle which include changes in how you eat, move, sleep and live. Understanding the purpose (your *why*) behind your goals will create a proactive approach to your fitness plan and a positive attitude towards embracing and pursuing new things in your life. This is the foundation to creating a healthier and active lifestyle. It will help you to overcome any challenges that come your way, and let's be honest, when life is busy those challenges will present themselves regularly.

CASE STUDY: TABITHA

Tabitha is a mum of three and an entrepreneur busy growing her business.[4] Her goal was to lose weight so that she would feel more confident within herself, as well as to get fitter and feel stronger so that she could have the energy to keep up with her kids and fully enjoy her time with them. This prompted her to start the transformation plan.

A few weeks into it she was finding it challenging to make improvements in her diet. We discovered that she was snacking a lot because she wasn't having proper meals during the day. I asked, 'OK, so what's stopping you from doing that?' She said that her time, energy and focus was on her work and kids and she had little for herself.

Although Tabitha had started her transformation plan, she found it challenging to embrace the new changes in her lifestyle. She needed someone to highlight her purpose to give her the motivation to create a positive change in her life. I asked her, 'What does it mean to you to lose weight? Why do you want to get fitter and stronger?' In that moment of honesty and vulnerability, she shared with me that it was important for her to look and feel better because of what she thought about herself. After having three children, her body had changed a lot and she wanted to get back to her pre-birth body, or as near to it as she could. She wanted to get stronger to reduce aches and pains and feel fitter so everyday activities didn't feel difficult.

4   Throughout the book I will be sharing real-life success stories of clients and their experiences. Many of the stories use real names while others are anonymous.

For her, losing weight meant to feel more confident and to get back to some sort of normality of how she looked, being stronger means to not feel pain and move better and feeling fitter is having the energy to run around with the kids and doing everyday physical activity with ease.

Recognising her purpose helped Tabitha to remember what it meant to her to look and feel better and that she needed to work on the first M (Mindset). In just two weeks she lost 2.5 kg (around 5.5 lbs), and with the wheels set in motion Tabitha continued to smash her goals and include exercise and healthy eating as part of her normal routine.

Your why

My question to you is: What's your why? Take a few minutes and ask yourself these questions:

- Am I happy with how I look and feel? (If not, why? Be honest.)

- What do I want to change and/or improve?

- What does it mean to me to achieve this?

- How will I feel when I achieve it?

- How will I feel if I don't achieve it?

- What could get worse?

Write down the answers on a piece of paper or type them on your phone because once you do that it becomes *real*, it's not just a thought or a feeling, it's something tangible that creates a shift in your mindset. This will channel your focus to achieve the results you really desire. Start to use the answers that you have in front of you: write them in your diary, use index cards, create a small poster, read them out loud and hear the words. Find whichever method works best for you. I find visualisation to be immensely powerful – harnessing the power of visualisation influences your actions, and your actions are the motion to manifest your goals to become a reality.

It's important to use whichever method works best for you because:

- It creates recognition. Recognising that you want to change or improve something (even if you knew it before) creates awareness, and that creates a conscious decision to do something about it (take action).

- Now you perceive a healthier lifestyle as more important because you have clarity of what you want to gain out of it. You know how you want to look and feel and what it means to you.

- This creates motivation, which is the accelerator to starting things. People don't suddenly think, 'Hmm, I need to exercise more,' or, 'I need to eat healthier.' There's generally something that prompts them to do it.

When you know your why, next on mindset is your beliefs. Let's look at what could be holding you back from achieving your goals and what you can do jump over those hurdles.

Your beliefs

Our beliefs can greatly influence the success or failure towards our path to looking and feeling great. They are so ingrained that it is only natural that they affect our wellbeing. Many of our beliefs are formed when we are children by accepting what others tell us to be true and our experiences in life. Other beliefs are analytically formed as we get older by examining them and determining whether they are true or not. Our set of beliefs helps us navigate through life.

Let's look at our beliefs about personal wellbeing – mainly exercise, diet and lifestyle choices. Throughout their lives most people have experienced different diets and types of exercise from what they've learned by having conversations with people, read, watched in the media and choices made by what they were willing to try at the time, yielding some successes and failures. During the time that you were trying and testing, you formed beliefs about what does and doesn't work for you. The question is, how do you know what is right for you?

Yes, one can learn from experience over time if something does or doesn't work for them, but if someone has constantly struggled to achieve their goals or has achieved them but keeps falling back to 'bad' habits, there's an underlying cause. That's where our beliefs come in. Our beliefs influence the choices we make; choices have a knock-on effect on our actions; actions performed with repetition and consistency over time become habits; and our habits reflect the results in different areas of our life. In my experience, most people don't follow a diet plan, exercise routine or a combination of the two rigorously. Research published in 2016 by *Patient Preference and Adherence* showed that 'a substantial proportion of people do not adhere to weight loss interventions.'[5] Why? Quite often the contributing factors are our levels of motivation at the time, focusing on other priorities, not being kept accountable and not having support and guidance to successfully adhere to a plan.

So how do you know if a diet or fitness plan has worked for you or not? There are a few answers to this question, but I would like you to consider the possibility that during those experiences limiting beliefs

---

5   M Lemstra et al, 'Weight loss intervention adherence and factors promoting adherence: A meta-analysis', *Patient Preference and Adherence*, 10 (2016), www.ncbi.nlm.nih.gov/pmc/articles/ PMC4990387/, accessed 30 March 2021

could have been formed which are now getting in your way.

CASE STUDY: MARIA

Maria is in her late forties. She has a young child and works full-time in the corporate world. She struggled to lose weight for many years and wanted to focus on having more energy to keep up with her child and long days at work and to lose weight to feel better about herself and feel good in her clothes. During her consultation, my question to her was, 'Why have you struggled to lose weight over the last ten years?' Maria replied frustratedly, 'I've tried diets before and they don't work for me, I just love my food.'

Maria had three limiting beliefs that were holding her back and she didn't even know it. Firstly, her belief that diets don't work. Secondly, her belief that her love of food was so great that she could not do without it. Thirdly, her belief that she'd been there and done that but nothing had worked.

By examining Maria's limiting beliefs together, Maria recognised them, accepted them and decided to work on them. I suggested that she focus on one challenge at a time – the first addressing her belief that diets don't work. Meals in the 5Ms talks about improving your diet rather than going on a diet, so rather than completely changing what Maria ate, I asked her to focus on how much she ate. Her first step was to improve her portion sizes by adopting personalised portions for protein, carbohydrates, fats and vegetables.

Within four weeks of consistently following the new and improved food portions, Maria lost a whole dress size – that's an incredible achievement considering she had battled with her weight for so long. The results changed her limiting belief of 'diets don't work' to one of 'it's better to improve my diet rather than going on a diet'. Maria continued to progress with her diet step by step by improving the food she ate. Her limiting belief that her love of food made it impossible for her to lose weight changed to 'I can have any food within a balanced diet' and her last belief that nothing worked changed to 'I needed to find what was right for me'.

Maria doubted that she would see any results due to her past experiences, but she started on the right foot and continued to commit to her plan. I encouraged her to put her previous experiences aside and it paid off. If she had continued to hold on to her limiting beliefs, she wouldn't have given the transformation plan a real go. Her results would not have been possible without first addressing her beliefs.

Limiting or negative beliefs prevent us from fulfilling our true potential and give rise to negative thoughts and emotions. Empowering our positive beliefs, on the other hand, allows us to act resiliently, believe in ourselves and invoke positive thoughts and emotions. Most people don't take the time to analyse them carefully and are not aware of their own beliefs, which can explain why some people thrive and succeed despite the most difficult circumstances while others fail.

To address your own beliefs, start by reflecting on past experiences when you tried to get fitter, lose weight or achieve any type of health and fitness goal. If you have never done a fitness plan but you currently have a goal to look and feel better, then think about what has led you to this point and if there are any beliefs that could have contributed. Once you have identified your limiting beliefs, if any, it is time to replace them with empowering ones. Pick a limiting belief and think about how that belief has held you back and worked against you. For example, let's say that your limiting belief is that you must finish what's on your plate – a belief most likely created in your childhood from parents who insisted you ate everything on your plate. Perhaps that has led you to overeat even when you're full.

Think of some specific examples of how this belief may have formed. Perhaps your mother got angry with you for not finishing your food, or your father rewarded you for finishing your food and you have fond memories of that, so you associate eating everything on your plate to be a good thing. Whether they're positive or negative experiences, they've created a limiting belief that you have followed throughout your life. This may have led to gaining weight or affected your previous experiences in trying to lose weight. Let the evidence sink in until you know in your heart and mind that your limiting belief was false. Really spend some time thinking about this until you know that it was not based on reality and you have the choice and power to change what you're doing for the better.

The next step is to replace your limiting or negative belief with an empowering and positive one. You could tell yourself, 'I don't have to finish everything on my plate.' Let go of your old belief, admit that it was false and limiting you, and start believing in your heart and your mind that there's nothing wrong with leaving food on your plate. The reality is that the food we eat should adequately satisfy our hunger and substantially nourish our body. Once we have had our fill of food, we don't need any more, we don't need to 'finish our plate' if we've eaten a healthy and balanced meal. By following this process, you are now more open to trying new things that can help you in your diet such as implementing the food portions like Maria did.

The last step is to be more mindful and have a little conversation with yourself if you see an old limiting belief surfacing. This is normal because our beliefs have been with us for so long and the thoughts and actions that follow them are on autopilot. Continuing with the example of the food portions – if you see yourself eating a meal and you feel satisfied, but you keep picking at the food left on your plate, recognise that moment and tell yourself, 'I feel good and don't need the rest of it.' It's these types of subtle reminders and conversations we have with ourselves that make the overall change, and this is empowering, especially when the results begin to show. The more you practise this, the sooner your subconscious mind will start inducing corresponding empowering thoughts, feelings and actions.

Take a moment to write down your thoughts on the following:

- What worked for me in my previous fitness plans?

- If any did work, do I maintain those results. If not, why?

- What didn't work?

- Do I perhaps have any beliefs that could be holding me back from looking and feeling great?

- What are my thoughts and feelings towards exercising?

- What are my thoughts and feelings towards food and my diet?

If you don't believe you have any limiting beliefs then you're ready to move on to the next chapter, but if you wrote something down it's time to reflect on your answers. Use them to complete the chart below and start creating empowering beliefs so that you can work on them and improve your quality of life. This can be a big breakthrough for people because it opens the doors to new possibilities, opportunities and experiences.

My current belief	I can't run/I'm not good at running.
Where it came from	Being slower than my classmates during PE classes at school.
Why it's not true	I haven't tried running again since I left school, so I don't know if I can do better with practice.
What I can do about it	• Start by going for a run without any goals of time, distance or calories burned, just to exercise, enjoy the outdoors, clear my mind and enjoy my favourite playlist. • Go running with friends for support and accountability. • Get a running coach to teach me how to run to build my skills and confidence.
My new beliefs	• I can run and even enjoy it. • Running helps me destress by having time for myself and enjoying the outdoors.

Focus on yourself

Prioritising yourself is the last phase of working on your mindset – it's about creating time and channelling your energy for you and just you. Creating some headspace from the busyness of life to clear your mind, reinvigorate your body and recharge.

Being a mother seldom leaves much freedom for you to do things for yourself and when life is busy there's never an ideal time to start a fitness routine. My point is that change can only happen when we choose for it to happen. You are responsible for your choices, it's down to you to focus your time and energy on yourself. Everyone I have worked with had made a conscious choice that something had to change, and they wanted to improve how they looked and felt about themselves. Yes, for some it was challenging making the commitment with their time, and some days felt harder than others, but they reached out for help to get support and guidance and followed through with the programme because it was important to them.

If you're unhappy with how you look and feel my advice is, *go for it*, make a change.

Whether you want to play sports, go to the gym, start taking classes or get a personal trainer, go for it. Whether you want to start drinking less or eating less sugar or eating more vegetables, go for it. I understand that right now you might be in a position where life feels a bit overwhelming, stressful and exhausting with everything going on, but with the right approach, it's feasible. If you're seeking some inspiration, I'd like to share the story of a client who had a good attitude and a positive approach to achieve her goals despite how hectic her life was.

CASE STUDY: JULIANNE

Julianne has three children and is a doctor at a London hospital. When we met, her work hours were intense. She was regularly on call (which meant she had to be available for emergencies), she did overtime and her shifts easily extended to twelve-hour days.

As if that wasn't enough, her husband was a doctor too. Add three children to the equation and it was a logistical nightmare, to say the least. If anyone had a good excuse not to start a fitness routine, Julianne did, but she really wanted to look and feel better and told herself, 'If I don't start now, I never will.' She had been contemplating exercising and eating better for over a year but didn't know where to start, so she reached out, and that's how we met.

During the consultation, I admired Julianne's 'can do' attitude. She started her transformation plan and in the first few weeks of focusing on herself, she found it surprisingly easy to incorporate the plan into her life. She was already seeing results in her body shape, she felt more energetic, her mood improved and she started sleeping better.

I asked her why she'd left it so long (it had been a few years since she'd exercised) and she said there had never been a good time, but she had finally chosen to do it anyway.

Many mothers feel they can't take time away from their kids and they are so focused on raising their children that they experience guilt when they do things for themselves. If you're feeling like this right now or you have experienced this before, I'm here to tell you that it's not selfish to look after yourself. It's a necessity, and I encourage you to do it. Start by making a conscious decision to focus on your food, exercise and making better lifestyle choices. If you're unsure of where to start or what to do, this book will provide you with the guidance you need.

2
Motivation

The second step in the 5Ms is Motivation. In this section you will discover why people succeed and fail in their fitness pursuits and how you can triumph in yours. Motivation is your reason (or reasons) for acting or behaving in a particular way. These reasons create actions, and actions will produce the results that you desire. Unfortunately, a lot of people don't have the motivation to exercise, eat healthier or commit to a fitness plan although they desire to look and feel great.

When I was a teenager, I was like the Michelin man (let's just say I had some extra weight). When I first started my fitness journey, I wasn't motivated to do anything, mainly because there were so many challenges that made it difficult for me to achieve my goal. At that age, many boys want to have a six-pack or big muscles, but for me, it was what I thought and felt about myself that drove me to start exercising, improve my diet and abandon old habits that held me back. Like so many others, I managed to find the motivation once my challenges were resolved, so let's start building up your motivation by jumping over those hurdles to create a clear pathway for you to get fitter, healthier and feel amazing. There are four main challenges that people commonly experience. I refer to them as TEAM: Time, Energy, Accountability, Mentorship.

Many people struggle with having little time for themselves, low energy levels, not having someone to keep them accountable and not having the guidance to know what to do. You may relate to some or all of these challenges. The good news is I'm going to show you how to overcome all of them.

Time

We spend most of our time on what we prioritise. For many people it's career/work, and parents have the added priority of raising their children. Let's use work as an example. We need money to pay our bills, fuel our lifestyles and have and do nice things. If you have a job that you love, it also nurtures your ambitions and gives meaning, purpose and fulfilment to your life. It's safe to say that for many, work is a priority – and rightly so, it has a lot of value. Children are another great example of how people spend and prioritise their time. Many parents would say the value that their children have on their lives and the profound love that they experience is indescribable. I'm blessed to have an amazing mother and as I've got older (and maybe even a little wiser), I've realised how much *time* she spent on me, the effort she put into raising me and the sacrifices she made. I thanked her for this recently and she replied, 'It's because I love you.' The moral of the story is that she always put me first and did everything for me – as do my clients for their children, and many other mothers. Quite often though, this results in neglecting their own needs, and at some point, many mothers reach a stage where they begin to feel frustrated or upset with how they look and feel about themselves and are ready for change.

If you want to look and feel better, whether that goal is to lose two dress sizes, to have more energy or to look amazing for a special day, you can make it happen, but you need to prioritise time for yourself to make that a reality. Imagine how great you will feel when you put on your favourite outfit and you're not wearing it, you *own* it – and so you should.

Let's take action and create time in your busy schedule. The 'me time' diary is a useful strategy to find pockets of time in your weekly schedule. The purpose of this exercise is to find time for yourself that you can commit to your food (Meals), exercise (Move) and healthy habits (Maximise).

Start by creating a weekly schedule on paper or your laptop and follow these steps:

- For those of you who work in a profession, block out your work time so you can focus on the time you do have available.

- For full-time mothers, block out work that routinely occupies your time.

- Whether you're at work or at home, highlight your lunchtime to eat a balanced meal and try to stick to it as much as possible (mums with newborns struggle with this more than others so don't worry if you're finding this challenging).

- Block out your time for everything children-related. Usually these are part of a routine: eg mealtime, bath-time, bedtime, school drop-off and pick-up, homework, after-school activities, weekend activities.

- Consider other children-related commitments such as chauffeuring, playdates and activities that tend to pop up week by week.

How much time do you have left for yourself? Let me guess – not much?

Firstly, I highly recommend outsourcing if you know someone that can do something better and faster – especially anything that you don't enjoy doing. This will free up your time to do the things you love and the things you're great at and give you more time to focus on yourself. Here are a few tips to free up your time at work, with children-related activities, and within the household:

- **Morning exercise:** Before everyone wakes up could be the perfect window to fit in your exercise. It doesn't need to be a long workout, even 20–30 minutes of moderate to high-intensity exercise such as high-intensity interval training (HIIT) is effective to burn a lot of calories and improve fitness. Within 45 minutes including shower and breakfast you're all done and ready for the day ahead.

- **Before dinner:** Children's routines are usually different to adults. If they eat and go to bed earlier than you, once the kids are in bed and before you sit down for dinner could be a good window to fit in your exercise. I appreciate you'll be feeling tired at this stage but if there isn't much choice elsewhere in your schedule this could be an option to consider.

- **During children's activities:** If you have more than one child, it's not uncommon for parents to split the kids up and take them to different activities. If you're outdoors in a park this could be a good opportunity to fit in a bodyweight workout (all you need is your exercise mat). If you're taking them to swimming classes and it's at a local gym, fitting in a quick class or burst in the gym is also an option.

- **Taking it in turns with your partner:** I've seen this work well for clients whether it's in the morning, evening or weekend. They both agree on a day and time they can commit to looking after the kids while their partner has their weekly dose of vitality. Everyone's schedule is different but try suggesting it – even if you both commit to it for a short period of time to get you kickstarted in your fitness routine, it will be beneficial.

- **Asking grandparents:** Most grandparents love looking after their grandchildren and if you're lucky to have your parents or in-laws nearby this is a great opportunity to leave the kids with them and get your exercise done. Having this type of social support can be helpful in committing to your fitness routine and achieving your goals.

- **Hiring a nanny:** If you don't already have a nanny this could be a great reason to have one. This will also give you more accountability to do your exercise because you have invested your time, energy and money for your health and fitness.

- **Playdates:** When you can leave your children with the other parents on the playdate these are great opportunities to have some time to fit in your exercise and/or have some time for yourself to recharge.

I know all the children-related activities are necessary and some you quite enjoy doing, but if you're limited for time and your diary doesn't look like it's changing any time soon, these are some options to consider when creating an exercise routine. I appreciate this can be harder if you're a single parent – based on my clients' experiences, the best options for them to find time to exercise have been in the mornings, asking grandparents, hiring a nanny or leaving their kids at a friend's house for a playdate.

Within the household, if you're doing everything for everyone else and you don't have enough time to focus on your needs, your goal is to get every child and adult that you currently do chores for to start doing their own. If the children are small this is easier because they are generally more compliant at this age and you can also turn tasks into a game, making it more fun for both of you. If they are older, you may get some resistance, but remind yourself of your need for time and also the importance of teaching them to be independent. Make a list of all the chores you do for others and start getting everyone to play their part. Here are a few examples:

- Get the children to tidy up their room well enough that you don't have to go over it again afterwards.

- Share the load of taking the bins out and replacing the old bin bags with new ones.

- Get everyone to clean up after themselves when they use the bathroom, shower and toilet.

- If you have pets, get someone to wash and brush the dog or go to the shops to buy cat food.

- Have someone help after dinner by washing the dishes or putting them away.

The list is endless, but you will know what's best for your household. The goal here is creating a balance between yourself, family and work.

The next challenge to consider is work. If you don't have any flexibility with how much time you spend on work then skip this part, but if your job involves meetings, keep reading. The main barrier my clients face at work is meetings. Working with CEOs, executives, managers and business owners, I have learned a thing or two about meetings, so here are a few options to consider:

- Do you need to be there? Free up some time by only going to the meetings you absolutely need to be present at.

- Does is it need to be a long meeting? Think about how much time you would save if you cut your meeting time by half or implemented fifteen-minute meetings. (There are many books, TED Talks and resources available on the effectiveness of short meetings.)

- Start and end meetings on time. If I had a penny for every client who cancelled their session because they were held up in a meeting, I'd be a millionaire. I recommend introducing highly productive and time-efficient meetings in your workplace. If you're in charge, I would start implementing these asap.

- Stop holding so many meetings.

Finally, try using the Eisenhower Matrix, which can be applied to any business. Eisenhower had to make tough decisions continuously about which of the many tasks he should focus on each day and this led him to invent the concept which helps us prioritise tasks by urgency and importance.[6] Identifying and prioritising your most important tasks can free up valuable time that you may be using on less important tasks, which can then either be delegated or don't need doing at all.

With your weekly 'me time' schedule ready by using the methods above you can see the remaining pockets of time left for yourself. Remember, if you don't have any time left for yourself to nurture your mind and body, it's a reflection of the choices you are making. I know sometimes some weeks are manic. That's inevitable and understandable, things can suddenly happen and your hands are tied – it's called *life*. I'm talking about your regular weekly routine that you do have control over and can now start shaping so you can look and feel better.

---

6   'Introducing the Eisenhower Matrix' (Eisenhower, no date), www. eisenhower.me/eisenhower-matrix, accessed 18 March 2021

To start adding exercise into your routine, choose how many times per week you can realistically commit to and create a fixed day and time for your exercise. This is optimal because you can automate it and doing so will give you the accountability to stick with it. If you can't create fixed times, then set a reminder to review your diary on a weekly basis and schedule your exercise. Exercising regularly should now start to feel more feasible, even if it means starting once per week and building it up from there. Next up is finding motivation when you don't have energy.

Energy

Everyone has experienced some form of tiredness which leaves them lacking in energy. You may resonate with some if not all of these forms of tiredness, and each (or even a combination) can create challenges for anyone who wants to get in shape:

- **Overdoing it:** Constantly pushing yourself and doing too much or more than is naturally healthy for you.

- **Tired and wired:** Finding it hard to switch off your mind (this can come from sleep deprivation or consuming too much caffeine).

- **Energy highs and lows:** Your energy levels fluctuate, leaving you feeling lethargic (from consuming too many sugary and caffeinated drinks and sugary snacks for a quick burst of energy).

- **Hollowness:** Constantly skipping meals leaves you running on an empty stomach and this can drop your energy levels.

- **Lack of stamina:** This can come from low iron levels, common among women who regularly experience heavy periods, during pregnancy or who are iron-deficient.

- **Decision fatigue:** The deterioration of your ability to make *good* decisions after a long session of decision-making. This reduces focus, willpower and your energy levels.

How many of those made you think, 'Yes, that's me'? Most mothers will say they've had all of them – sometimes all at once. Typically, a lack of energy leads to a lack of motivation. Being tired negatively affects your decision-making and you're most likely to make decisions with the least amount of resistance. Usually these aren't the best ones to help you look and feel better. How often have you had a sleepless night and told yourself, 'I fancy doing a workout,' the next day? If you have then I applaud you, but most of us just want to curl up on the sofa and doze off.

So, what can be done about starting or maintaining a fitness routine when you are constantly tired? You will find your motivation to exercise, eat healthier and have good habits in your life by following one rule: *Make it simple.* If it's not simple, it will not work, period. There is already so much complexity in life and you don't need your fitness routine to add to that. It needs to be integrated into your lifestyle and not feel like a chore.

CASE STUDY: BETHANY

A good example of why simplicity works is when I worked with Bethany. She was in her fifties, had a child starting secondary school and was a senior manager at her workplace. At the time she was feeling stressed and overwhelmed at work, her son was going through a rebellious phase and she was experiencing menopause. She felt exhausted every day.

To begin with, we did regular sessions every week to build momentum and create a foundation in her fitness routine, but she still felt tired because her work and home life didn't change. Bethany felt that the exercise and improving her diet were additional tasks to her day and this wasn't sustainable. We talked about making things easier and simpler to do and make this part of her lifestyle. Bethany knew that if she didn't do a little bit of planning and prepping for the week ahead then it wouldn't work. It's difficult to face little but significant barriers such as not having the right food available or not scheduling your workout when you are tired – a molehill can seem like a mountain. We've all experienced this before: by making things simple, you are better prepared. Bethany began to order her food shopping online every Thursday evening so that she had her (and her family's) food ready for the following week. This meant it was easy to make healthy food choices because they were available. She took the same approach with her exercise by using the 'me time' diary to commit time for exercise every week and had someone to keep her accountable to it.

Bethany had clarity on what to do and how to do it, which helped her make better choices, especially when she was tired. This was down to following the golden rule: make it simple. During her transformation plan she lost 9 kg (that's more than a dress size). She felt good in her clothes, which made her happier, she had more energy throughout the day, and she was proud of her achievement, which built her confidence in her appearance.

Here are five ways to make exercise and eating healthier easier:

- Choose a physical activity with the fewest reasons or excuses not to do it (some will need accountability, which I'll be discussing in the next section).

- Plan your food shopping in advance to have the meals and snacks that are in alignment with your fitness goal so when you're feeling tired and hungry you have the right food on hand.

- Schedule your weekly exercise in advance and commit to it.

- Avoid overwhelming yourself with unrealistic tasks by focusing on small daily improvements such as improving what you eat and drink, how much exercise you do, increasing your downtime, etc.

- Have a mentor to guide, support and motivate you (you will find out more about this in the following chapter).

Accountability

Accountability is immensely powerful and will be a great asset to your fitness journey. It helps you to define your goals, empowers you, encourages personal excellence, creates a better support network and strengthens your success in achieving your results. To create a fitness routine that seamlessly fits into your life it's important to find out what type of method is going to benefit you the most. In everyday life, when we need to resolve a problem or complete a task there are three ways to do it:

- DIY: Do It Yourself
- DIWY: Do It With You (you do it with someone)
- DIFY: Do It For You (someone does it for you)

There are various factors that will influence your choice of method, but the four main decision-makers are importance, time, money and commitment. In this case, the problem is someone struggling to lose weight. Let's say the goal is to lose 10 kg.

The first option (DIY) means you buy a general, ready-made fitness plan at a low cost. It does what it says on the tin – you do everything yourself: the background research in finding a suitable fitness plan, choosing a plan you believe is good for you and committing to the workouts and the diet until you achieve your 10-kg weight-loss goal. This involves 100% of your commitment and self-discipline to stay accountable and motivated throughout the duration of the plan to see results. This option is perfect for anyone who is self-motivated and has the time and energy to do their workouts and commit to their eating plan. If the idea of achieving your fitness goal on your own doesn't faze you, and you don't mind some trial and error to see whether it's going to work or not, because it's a generalised rather than tailored plan, then this is an option for you. The DIY method is for anyone who wants a low-cost fitness solution to which they are happy to commit 100% of their effort.

The second option (DIWY) is doing it with health and fitness professionals such as nutritionists, dieticians, personal trainers, coaches, etc. This option is perfect for anyone who wants to achieve their goal but can't do it alone and wants someone to give them everything they need to follow. It still requires a level of commitment and self-discipline but only to an extent compared to being on your own because you have maximum accountability, guidance and motivation throughout your fitness journey. The benefit of working one-on-one is that it's personalised, so there's minimal trial and error. Your diet is tailored, your exercise plan is suited for your body and fitness levels and the one-on-one support helps you overcome your challenges by having someone there to guide you. People choose this option when they want a service that delivers faster and safer results and want a guarantee that their time, energy and money is put to the best use. The DIWY option is for anyone who wants a medium-cost fitness solution which they can commit to with support, guidance and accountability from a professional with maximum results.

The third option (DIFY) is the 'high cost with instant results' option. In this scenario, it's liposuction. I'm not for or against cosmetic surgery – this is a personal choice – so let's look at the pros and cons and who might choose this. This is for anyone who wants to lose weight in one go without having to exercise, improve their diet or change certain lifestyle choices. The cosmetic surgeon will tell you how much body fat they can safely remove before the procedure is performed. It doesn't require any self-discipline or commitment to do, but it comes at a high cost and you have to be comfortable with the idea of having surgery and the recovery process that comes with it.

You might be thinking, 'Hmm, not much effort and quick results?' If you want to go down this route, bear in mind that an experienced professional surgeon will recommend that you eat a healthy diet and exercise regularly to maintain the results. The reality is that the vast majority of people gain weight due to their lifestyle choices. That won't change in one day, even if you're a few kg lighter. It takes time to change those habits and adopt a new mindset as to how you live your life, so even the DIFY option requires commitment and discipline after your surgery to maintain it. If you don't, it will all go back on, which encourages the idea of implementing a healthier lifestyle in the first place. This is one of many reasons why I don't think liposuction is the best choice – I genuinely believe that you can naturally lose weight, look great and feel incredibly good about yourself with exercise, a healthy diet and good habits.

Accountability greatly increases your chances of achieving a goal. Think of a time when you turned up for an appointment because you didn't want to let the other person down, even though that appointment was for your benefit, or when someone booked an appointment with you and needed your accountability and how much they benefited from it. Many of us care more about not letting other people down than letting ourselves down. When it comes to your fitness plan this is not a bad thing because it's a powerful driver to keep you committed to your plan.

Picture the positive impact it would have if you regularly checked in with a nutrition coach for your diet or had a personal trainer ready at your home, workplace or gym. Think of all those mornings when you wanted to exercise but didn't have the motivation to because you were just too tired, or when you got home from work and the intention to exercise was there but it was too much of a struggle to motivate yourself. With someone there to keep you accountable you don't need to find the motivation. It takes out the whole thinking process too – you just do it. It's this type of consistency that create results. Going to exercise classes is also effective, but finding the right class is important because it's the spirit of community within that class that creates good accountability. How do you find the right one? Try them and see what works for you.

Accountability encourages personal excellence, because you acknowledge responsibility for the foods you eat, the need to include exercise in your routine, and how far you have progressed towards your fitness goals. This is great because it establishes awareness to implement those changes but adhering to them is the challenge, so having a support network that can keep you accountable is useful.

Having accountability will help you to clearly define your goals. If you want to be held accountable for your actions as you attempt to reach your goal, you need to be specific. For example, 'I want to be smaller,' can be replaced with, 'I want to lose a dress size in three months.' 'I want to lose weight,' can be replaced with, 'I want to lose 7 kg by the end of June for our summer holiday.' Setting a specific goal and tracking it will greatly improve your motivation levels and chances of reaching your fitness goals because you have clarity and a timeframe, so when you tell your fitness buddy, personal trainer or community, they know what to hold you accountable to.

Clearly defining your goals builds motivation because you know what you want. Remember to think of your *why*: why do you want it? To strengthen your chances of success, share details of what you want to achieve and your progress in a public way. This can be with your family, friends, a fitness buddy, personal trainer, work colleagues or the community of people in your fitness class or sports group. Sharing makes it become *real*. The key is to make the people in your life aware of your goal and your progress towards it. If you manage to reach that goal, it will increase your perceived status and respectability among the people around you, which is a positive psychological motivator. If you fail to reach the goal, you may feel shame and a loss of respect, which is a powerful negative motivator that you will work hard to avoid. These kinds of negative motivators are especially useful when you want to achieve something that is meaningful to you. It's often a fear of failure that gives us more determination and drive.

When you tell people about your fitness goals, they will also usually be supportive and begin to actively help you reach those goals. For example, if your friends and family know you are trying to lose weight, they won't offer you unhealthy foods and they might decide to change their eating habits. Your work colleagues will be less likely to offer you cakes and snacks if they know you are improving your diet and have a goal to achieve.

CASE STUDY: YVONNE

Yvonne was struggling to lose weight due to a combination of working long hours and raising her child. One of her main challenges was eating too much sugar – she relied on it for energy throughout the day to power her through work and keep up with her little one at home. She felt addicted to it.

Simply telling Yvonne to stop eating sugar or giving her healthier alternatives was not going to cut it. She needed accountability to give her the motivation to start doing something about it and keep her committed to follow through with it, so I proposed a seven-day commitment to eating healthier. During those seven days, Yvonne had to send me a picture of all her meals, snacks and everything she drank throughout the day.

What happened? Yvonne upped her game. By having to send me the pictures she automatically became more mindful of her food choices because she didn't want to send me pictures of a chocolate muffin at work and a slice of fireman Sam cake at the weekend birthday party. The cake became a square of dark chocolate and the muffin was replaced by a piece of fruit. Yvonne continued the seven-day commitment to eat healthier for twelve weeks and combined with exercise she lost a total of 10 kg.

Yvonne was so happy with her results – she'd been meaning to do it for a while, and she finally had. It was a great accomplishment, with a big part of her success due to being held accountable to someone.

I've personally benefited from accountability. I used to be a nervous flyer and it was gradually getting worse, so one day I thought to myself, 'If I jump out of a plane, I won't be scared to be sat in one.' A bit of an odd theory perhaps, but that's what came to mind. That same day I did a social media post telling everyone that my lovely wife, Lily, and I were skydiving for charity in seven days' time. Now I had maximum accountability. Being totally honest, I was excited when I did the post, but I felt pure fear afterwards – the fear of jumping out of that plane became so real. I even had trouble sleeping for a few nights. I thought to myself, 'Michael, what on earth have you just done?' People started donating money for a charity dedicated to a family member of mine who was ill at the time. Now it had become more than just me facing my fears – it was about a bigger cause and purpose. This kept me accountable to my promise of skydiving.

It was a beautiful Saturday morning. The sky was clear blue and the sun was shining. I was sitting on the edge of a propeller plane looking down from 10,000 feet, attached to the instructor behind me. We rocked back and forth ready to jump on the count of three, but you know they always do it at two, and off we went. That moment was the most liberating and exhilarating experience I've ever had, and I managed to do it because I didn't want to let myself down, and I certainly didn't want to let everyone else down. That's the power of accountability. (By the way, I'm good on planes now. It worked.)

Now that you know how effective it is to have someone keep you accountable, ask yourself these questions:

- Do I know what fitness routine is right for me?

- Do I have the motivation to exercise alone?

- Can I commit to a healthier eating plan on my own?

If any of your answers are no, then I encourage you to seek guidance and find some form of accountability to achieve your goal of looking and feeling great.

Mentorship

There are several things that most people find challenging when working to achieve their health and fitness goals. First, it's finding the motivation to exercise and eat a balanced diet. Second, it's not knowing what to do. Third, it's being consistent with it all. Many struggle to maintain their fitness routine and need guidance and accountability to be consistent. I'm going to show you how having a mentor can help you overcome these challenges and the benefits of having one during various stages in your life.

There are three stages when mothers experience what I term the 3Cs: Change, Challenge and Comeback. The first is pregnancy (pre- and postnatal), the second is family life and the third is menopause. Each stage interconnects with the others and has its own set of challenges, so having a mentor offering guidance during each stage is a highly effective way to stay fit and healthy, and lose weight, if that's the goal.

Pregnancy

As nature takes its course during those nine months, it is normal to experience hormonal, physical, emotional and psychological changes. It's important to stay active, to move well, stay strong and improve your daily life by having the strength to meet the demands of a growing child. A 2016 study showed that 'a physical exercise program during pregnancy is associated with a shorter first stage of labor'.[7] Other benefits of exercise during pregnancy include:

- Faster recovery after childbirth

- Better mood and energy levels

- Improved sleep

- Reduced pregnancy discomfort (backache, leg cramps, bloating, swelling, etc)

---

7   M Perales et al, 'Regular exercise throughout pregnancy is associated with a shorter first stage of labor', *American Journal of Health Promotion* (2016), https://journals.sagepub.com/doi/pdf/10.4278/ajhp.140221-QUAN-79, accessed 30 March 2021

- Improved odds of maintaining a healthy weight

- A lower risk of gestational diabetes

The number one question pregnant women ask before exercising is, 'Is this safe to do?' That's their ultimate worry and a lot of women don't exercise during their pregnancy because of fear of the unknown. By having the right mentor with the appropriate qualifications and experience working with prenatal clients, you will benefit from a safe and effective fitness plan that will keep you strong throughout your pregnancy. When I'm working with prenatal clients, I adapt their plans accordingly for each trimester by taking a holistic approach encompassing sleep, stress, nutrition, exercise and movement.

As you move back into your normal routine after birth, the focus is to strengthen your core area, which will have a positive impact on your posture, body movements, strength and fitness levels. The main exercises to start with are lower abdominal, pelvic floor, glute activation exercises and walking for the cardio benefits. Postnatal exercises are important and help by:

- Reducing aches and pains

- Assisting with weight loss if pursued with a balanced diet

- Enhancing stamina levels to cope with the demands of a newborn

- Toning your body and increasing muscle strength

Once you have recovered from the initial few weeks of giving birth, I strongly recommend you work with a pre- and postnatal qualified fitness coach (mentor) to kickstart your fitness routine and benefit from the advantages of exercise.

Family life

This book is predominantly based on how to look and feel great during this phase because it's the longest stage out of the three. It is also during this stage that people experience the most challenges such as lack of time, feeling tired, stressed and not motivated to do a fitness plan alone. Stress from work, family and an accumulation of life itself can feel exhausting and overwhelming, so having a mentor during this time is hugely beneficial. Whenever you face an obstacle to achieving your goal, your mentor can give you the solution. When you're having an off day, they are there to listen and provide guidance. Little things like sending a text to see how you're progressing and sending reminders to keep you on track with your food and keep you accountable with doing your exercise are also helpful. All of this can make a difference between success or failure in achieving your goal of looking and feeling better.

The reason why people choose to have someone to help them is that they want to take the thinking process out of losing weight, getting in shape or any goal they have. They want someone to tell them what to do, how to do it and when to do it to get the results they want. How great would it be if you knew exactly what to do and you just did it rather than going through all the guesswork, trying and failing, or not doing anything at all for years because of procrastination or simply not knowing what to do?

Data collected from 500 women who had one-to-one training consultations with BrigoPT showed that their goals, challenges and priorities were all similar. They commonly expressed that their focus during family life was looking after themselves, getting back into shape, losing weight and feeling better inside and out overall. This is easier to achieve with a bit of help. Let's be honest – trying to get in shape can be challenging on the best of days, even without kids or a demanding job. Adding those to the equation can make it feel nearly impossible. On a separate note, you're also setting an example and being a role model to your children when living a healthier lifestyle. It shows the importance of taking care of yourself when you exercise, eat healthy food and make positive lifestyle choices. This can certainly inspire and rub off on them in the future.

Menopause

Menopause is a highly individual experience, and its effects vary from woman to woman. One common effect is weight gain – many women find that their weight has crept up or they have suddenly gained weight due to menopause, and for many, the weight has shifted to their stomach area. There are a number of factors which influence this, including hormonal changes, aging, lifestyle and genetics. We're going to look at the best approaches to get in shape during the three transitions of menopause and why it's beneficial to have a mentor during this time.

Perimenopause

This is the stage when the body begins the transition – women start at different ages, some as early as thirties but typically it's in the forties. During this time hormones are changing, oestrogen levels become erratic and progesterone levels decline. This can influence weight and may lead to weight gain. In one study, levels of ghrelin (often referred to as the 'hunger hormone') were found to be significantly higher among perimenopausal women compared to pre- and postmenopausal women.[8] High levels of ghrelin could mean a person finds themselves feeling hungry even if they haven't done much physical activity.

With correct guidance and support from a mentor, knowing how to adjust your diet is a great benefit in preventing any further weight gain and promoting a healthier and more active lifestyle. Your metabolism is at a low phase and it will require more effort to lose

---

8   MR Sowers et al, 'Change in adipocytokines and ghrelin with menopause', *Maturitas*, 59/2 (2008), www.maturitas.org/article/ S0378-5122(08)00003-0/fulltext, accessed 30 March 2021

weight, primarily through a healthy diet. What you can do right now is to have smaller, healthy food portions by following the hand portion method for each food group (carbohydrates, proteins, fats, and vegetables) in each meal. The method is explained in full in Step 3 of the 5Ms (Meals). Fats are essential to keep your taste buds happy, so rather than avoiding them to get in shape, assess the types of fats you're eating. Vegetable fats such as extra-virgin olive oil, coconut oil, nuts, seeds and avocado (technically a fruit) are the healthiest form – include these in your diet using the hand portion method to keep those calories in check.

It's also important to consider that this transition is occurring during the family life stage, so if you do gain weight, it's likely due not only to hormones but also to lifestyle. Hormonal changes can certainly make it more challenging to get in shape, but it's good news to know that lifestyle is a big factor as you have the power to influence that. The sooner you start making these lifestyle changes, the more you can benefit in the following transitions and later life.

During menopause

Menopause usually occurs in the early fifties. Not everyone experiences weight gain, but many women do notice changes in their body shape. What's happening is that their body composition is changing: muscle mass decreases and body fat increases without much change to weight, but the body shape becomes visibly different. People are also generally less active than when they were younger, which reduces energy expenditure and leads to a loss of muscle mass. This is a good reason to have the right mentors around you to provide the best exercise for fitness, strength and calorie burn. Adjusting your diet to eat foods that are nutritionally rich but lower in calories will also help you to lose a healthy amount of weight.

To get in shape and improve health it's best to include a combination of resistance exercise to strengthen and tone the body with cardiovascular exercise for increased energy levels, cardio benefits and added calorie burn. This combination will give you a well-rounded fitness plan and provide better results in how you look and feel.

Postmenopause

This starts after one year has passed since your last menstrual cycle. Some symptoms may continue but it's common for them to subside at this stage. Living an active lifestyle and being mindful of what you eat is a must if you want to stay strong, have energy and feel good. If you have a goal to achieve, having a mentor to show you how to achieve it is an excellent starting point. Later in the book I'll share a success story of Joanne, who achieved great results in her postmenopausal years.

Key benefits of having a mentor

- You will benefit from a safe exercise plan during pregnancy to keep you strong and fit to carry the weight of the baby, and the added benefits of a shorter labour.

- It cuts out the thinking process of losing weight during the family life stage. Having a mentor can help make looking and feeling better during this somewhat hectic phase a reality.

- It will help you achieve your goals during any menopausal stage by knowing what to do and having the correct guidance.

3
Meals

The third step in the 5Ms is Meals. Diet is an important element to consider and if your goal is to look better, tone up or lose weight, there's a degree of fat loss involved. I'm going to show you why improving your diet is preferable to and easier than going on a diet, a simple but effective method for naturally reducing calories by tweaking your food portions, why improving food quality is important, how you can use food services to fast-track results, and the effects of emotional eating.

The word diet comes from the Greek *diaita*, which means 'a way of life'. I love that. A way of life. That's what a diet should be, but it's perceived differently. Most people associate the word diet with words like boring, bland, difficult, restrictive and unrealistic.

They think of eating carrots and celery sticks, doing a juice 'cleanse' or eliminating carbs. Just writing it down feels depressing. No wonder nobody likes diets. There is often a media craze accompanying a new, trendy (crash) diet, whether it's low-carb, low-fat, fruit only or drinking vinegar – you name it, it exists. There are even diets followed by entire communities of people who swear by them.

Why diets seldom work

When have you ever seen anyone jumping for joy when they've had to go on a diet? Here are a few reasons why many people don't like diet plans and why they often don't work:

- They are too restrictive.

- They are difficult to maintain, so not sustainable in the long term.

- They are mentally tiring (ie they involve calorie counting, weighing food, crunching numbers every day).

- They are difficult to follow in sociable environments (restaurants, eating at a friend's house, parties, etc).

- They require a lot of motivation and self-discipline.

- They create an unhealthy relationship with food.

- They eliminate a certain food group or groups, which can deprive you of vital nutrients.

- Dieting is part of the 'thin ideal' – people believe they need to diet to be slim.

Rigid diet plans can and usually do go wrong. Do any of the following scenarios ring a bell?

You follow the plan for a little while but you're feeling miserable

Why? You miss out on social events to avoid the temptation of breaking your diet, you don't feel good, you're not happy and it's just not sustainable. Diet plans expect you to completely change your habits and lifestyle in one go. That takes an incredible amount of motivation and self-discipline and it's a huge amount of change – it's stressful, overwhelming and not at all enjoyable.

You don't stick to the plan

You're feeling motivated and enthusiastic at the start, but a few days or weeks in, you find it's just too tough to follow. Life gets in the way because you're busy, not always prepared, your boss expects you to work late, kids get sick and sometimes you just don't feel like having an apple and kale super-smoothie at 8am. The motivation has plummeted and you're back to old habits again.

You follow the plan too well and for too long

Most diet plans are meant to be temporary. They're designed to help a person achieve a specific, short-term goal like dropping a few extra kg before a wedding or a holiday. Eventually, you realise it's not sustainable and revert to your previous diet, and for most people that normally leads to putting weight back on or not shifting it at all.

It's too technical

Some diets may say, 'Eat protein throughout the day, carbs only in the afternoon and vegetables at night.' OK, but what's considered a protein or a carbohydrate? Some diets focus exclusively on nutrients or measurements, which can become confusing. We rarely measure our daily meals precisely (casseroles, pasta dishes, salads, etc). We know the recipes well, so we don't think, 'An ounce of this, 200 grams of that, a teaspoon of this…'

Improving your diet

If you want to eat better, it doesn't need to be complicated. You simply need to use the golden rule: *make it simple.* You don't need to weigh, measure and track everything or count every calorie. People who do this are generally paid to be in optimal shape as part of their profession. If you're not being paid to do this then you don't really need to follow this type of approach. Instead, you need to think about what you're already eating and how you could make it a little bit better. This means adjusting your current diet, which involves making small changes and improvements to what you already normally eat and enjoy, one small step at a time.

What do the most successful diets have in common? They:

- Are low in added and artificial sugar

- Eliminate refined carbohydrates

- Eliminate trans fats

- Are high in vegetables and fibre

- Focus on *food* instead of calories

These factors indicate food quality, and this is what you should focus on instead of choosing the trendiest or most popular diet. To avoid choosing a diet plan that's not right for you, the above factors are geared towards optimal health. Optimal health also means ideal body weight, so if your goal does include losing weight then applying these factors will certainly help in achieving that goal.

There are also other factors which we're going to go through in the next few pages to create a well-rounded, balanced diet designed for anyone who wants to look and feel great. Then you can implement 'a way of life' approach by improving your current diet to make it part of your lifestyle, whether you want to lose or maintain weight, get in shape, have more energy or experience optimal health.

Rather than thinking about bad or good foods, think of a range of food quality. In each meal the intention is to *make this meal just a little bit better* in every situation. Let's use breakfast as the example. Here's how improving it step by step might look in daily life:

Stage 1: You've got to get the kids ready for school. Time flies and you're rushing out the door, so you pick a whipped-cream coffee drink and croissant on your way into work, wolfing it down while you're driving.

Now your game is to improve your breakfast just a little bit, starting with what you already have or do.

Stage 2: You've rushed out the door, but you replace the croissant with a whole-grain muffin. Instead of a 'dessert in a cup', you get a regular coffee with single cream and sugar. You grab a yoghurt on your way out of the house for a bit of protein. You're still rushed and busy, but you eat your breakfast while scrolling through emails at work which is a good start. Well done.

Now we're stepping up our game.

Stage 3: You switch the muffin to granola with cottage cheese or Greek yoghurt. You switch the cream in your coffee for 2% milk. You add some colourful fruit. You're now eating out of your plate on a table instead of takeaway packages in the car. You're checking out the news while you eat.

Now you're at pro level.

Stage 4: You change 'rushing and panicked' to 'set aside a little extra time to enjoy a leisurely breakfast'. You cleverly prep an omelette with veggies in advance on your food prep day. You reduce your coffee or change it to green tea since you've noticed that too much coffee was tweaking you out. The protein plus colourful fruit and veg have become the stars of the meal. You discover you like hot lemon water. (What? Is this really me?) You eat mindfully, feeling relaxed, while having a few minutes to yourself, maybe even watching the sunrise.

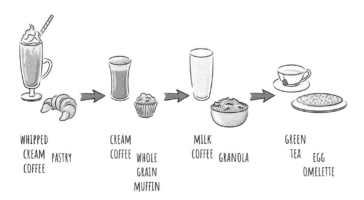

WHIPPED CREAM PASTRY COFFEE

CREAM COFFEE WHOLE GRAIN MUFFIN

MILK COFFEE GRANOLA

GREEN TEA EGG OMELETTE

You have just shifted from being on a diet plan that's restrictive, unsustainable and pretty miserable, to one where you have choices and variety while dropping a dress size or two. Improving your meals is about making them better – there's no need to be perfect. You decide how far you need to progress along the food stages. It depends on what *you* want, what *you* need and what *you* can reasonably do right now. Things can also change over time – it's your choice. There are several benefits of following this approach:

- No more suffering with fad diets

- No more yo-yo dieting

- Enjoy food while losing weight

- Be social and enjoy occasions without worrying about breaking your diet

- See fast but, most importantly, lasting results

Most people have the impression that getting in shape needs to be difficult (remember the 'no pain, no gain' proverb?), but it doesn't need to be. I'm not saying it won't require effort and commitment, because it will, but this approach will reduce frustration, confusion and struggle. This is also not a race to lose the largest amount of weight in the quickest time. This is what most people want when they go on a diet, and usually it comes back on anyway. Don't worry – weight loss will happen. You don't need to lose sight of losing weight, but also focus on improving the way you live to make the whole process more enjoyable. In doing so, you will look and feel great.

CASE STUDY: KATHRYN

If it sounds too good to be true, let me tell you about Kathryn. When we first met, she didn't exercise at all and her diet consisted of high-calorie foods and fast food. With a combination of entertaining clients and being extremely social, there was also a lot of drinking involved, with the added weekend binges. Kathryn used to make sudden and drastic changes to her eating by going on various diets, but this approach wasn't working for her.

I suggested she tried a different approach and improve her current diet. Kathryn embraced the changes in her diet by reducing fast food and alcohol, making better food choices and eating appropriate portions. It's what I call a lifestyle diet. She put in the effort to improve each meal week by week until she had reached a balance of achieving her weight loss goal while simultaneously enjoying life. This was a diet that she could maintain, and which fitted in well with her life. She found it mentally easier and more realistic than completely cutting out a certain food group (eg a diet where you can't eat carbohydrates). Instead, she reduced certain foods or switched to others that were better for her goal. This was sustainable for Kathryn and it worked beautifully. She still went out with friends and enjoyed social occasions, but she made good food decisions.

With the combination of regular strength and cardiovascular exercise, Kathryn lost an incredible

4 stone (that's 25.4 kg or 56 lbs), equivalent to over three dress sizes. She felt amazing and was so happy with her results. She looked stunning. We've continued to stay in contact over the years and I'm pleased to say she has maintained her results and her healthier lifestyle.

An ideal diet is one that works for you, not one that you have to work for. Yes, you need to put effort into eating healthier, but your diet must work around your lifestyle rather than you having to manage your lifestyle around your diet. Think of your diet as two circles – a small circle within a big circle. Now imagine a dancer practising a dance routine. For her to become the best that she can be, she needs to learn how to dance within the small circle, but sometimes she steps out of it into the bigger circle. As she gets better and keeps practising, she dances within the small circle more often.

The small circle contains the foods that are good for you: for your health, beauty, vitality and longevity. The big circle contains the food and drinks that you enjoy having but which aren't in alignment with your goals. If you have too many or too much of these foods or beverages, they will slow you down or even stop you from looking and feeling better. You will occasionally step into the big circle, and that's OK; it's normal, so don't beat yourself up for it. What is important is that you choose to step back into the small circle and continue progressing towards your goal. This way you can enjoy life, have more balance and stick to a sustainable diet which is *your* diet.

Key points to remember:

- Don't go on a prescribed diet – improve your current one.

- Focus on improving one meal at a time until all your meals are optimal for your goals and your lifestyle.

- Your diet must be sustainable to see any weight loss results and to keep the weight off.

- The key ingredient is consistency. Be consistent with improving your meals until it becomes normal for you.

- Enjoy the process. It's a change at first, but you will quickly adapt to it.

Portion sizes

Now that you know how to approach your diet by focusing on improving it, the next progression is having the correct food portions to give you energy, promote weight loss and not leave you starving. Finding the right food portions is one of the simplest and most successful strategies to improve your diet and lose weight, but calorie counting can be annoying and impractical and having to crunch numbers every day can lead to frustration, which reduces adherence to a healthier eating plan. It is also quite often inaccurate.

There's a better way to get the correct portion and balance of food at every meal: all you need is your hand. This strategy means you don't need to weigh food, count calories or keep track of everything (although a food diary does have its benefits). The reason why so many clients have found this useful is because of its simplicity. Your hand is proportionate to your body, its size never changes and it always with you, making it the perfect tool for measuring. This is how it works:

- For protein, it's your palm size.

- For carbohydrates, it's your cupped hand.

- For fats, it's your thumb size.

- For vegetables, it's your fist size (equivalent to a handful).

This is a meal portion specific to you.

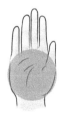
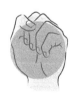
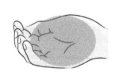
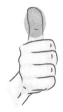

A SERVING OF PROTEINS = 1 PALM

A SERVING OF VEGETABLES = 1 FIST

A SERVING OF CARBS = 1 CUPPED HAND

A SERVING OF FATS = 1 THUMB

This versatile method can be used anytime and anywhere, so whether you're out for dinner, ordering a work lunch or at home, you know how much to eat. When you're not in control of your food choices (let's say you're at a friend's house for a weekend lunch), you don't need to worry about breaking your diet and feeling guilty because you can control the amount of food you eat. This is not the case with other diets (eg low-fat diets, low-carb diets or diets with fixed eating times), which make it difficult to enjoy yourself when you're out. Simply follow the hand portion guide with options served at the social setting you're in. Of course, it requires a degree of discipline, but that's fair seeing as you're not restricting yourself from anything; you are simply having less of it, which comes in handy (excuse the pun).

How quickly you adjust to the hand portions approach will vary from person to person, but I'm going to fast-track it for you by explaining what to expect at the start. For the first few days you will be learning how much of each food group you can eat in one meal so you will need to use your hand or a cup to measure it out. Eventually you will have a good visual cue of what an ideal plate looks like and can apply this to any meal.

You can either gradually apply the hand portions to one meal at a time (eg focus on improving your food portions for dinner each day and then work your way through lunches and breakfasts, until you've adjusted every meal in every day), or you can start on every meal straight away. There's no right or wrong approach: some people like to dive right in while others need to do it step by step. Choose what works for you until you can stick to it consistently.

It is normal to feel hungry for the first few days – your stomach needs to adjust to the new portion sizes, after all. How hungry you will feel will depend on how much you are eating right now, the amount of food you're eating in one sitting and the type of food you're eating. The good news is the human body is incredible at adapting and your body will soon get used to it.

One of the many benefits my clients have experienced is a reduction in appetite. This approach regulated their appetites and even reduced the amount of sugar they consumed. This is due to balancing blood sugar levels, and when people control their food portions, they also make better food choices, thereby reducing food cravings that usually come from high-fat and high-carb foods. This is a big win for anyone who wants to lose weight. Stick with it and before you know it this way of eating will become your new normal.

CASE STUDY: SARAH

I remember introducing this approach to Sarah. She had a newborn boy and all her time was committed to raising him. Even cooking a meal can be difficult when children are that age, so I suggested that she focus on how much she ate rather than what she ate. Within a few weeks she had lost 2 kg. That's how effective reducing your portions is. Because Sarah was mindful of her portions, she had better awareness of her food choices and quickly improved what she ate. Combined with her new food portions, this became a powerful combination to losing more weight.

Sarah continued to improve her diet in all areas, and combined with regular exercise, she achieved her goal to lose 7 kg. She was so happy with her results and felt like herself again.

The hand portion method is not dissimilar to traditional eating behaviours in Japan. Culturally, they have a healthy attitude to food and eating which is taught from a young age. They have a saying, *'hara hachi bu'*, which means to eat until you are 80% full. The way the Japanese serve their food is also key. Rather than having one large plate, they often eat from a small bowl and several different dishes, usually a bowl of rice, a bowl of miso, some fish or meat and then two or three vegetables dishes, often served communally and eaten in rotation. This certainly provides food for thought – the Japanese have one of the lowest levels of obesity among developed countries worldwide.[9] It's more challenging to be slimmer and healthy in a developed country because food is often more bountiful, and we have many options to choose from. Smaller food portions and healthy food choices have multiple health benefits.

---

9   'OECD obesity update 2017' (OECD, 2017), www.oecd.org/health/obesity-update.htm, accessed 20 May 2021

To get you started, here is an example of an ideal plate:

- For protein, it's a palm-sized chicken breast.

- For carbohydrates, it's a cupped handful of whole-grain rice.

- For vegetables, it's a fist-sized portion (equivalent to a handful) of mixed vegetables such as carrots, peas and green beans.

- For fats, it's a thumb-sized amount of extra-virgin olive oil to put over the veggies as a condiment.

That's what your plate will look like. When you're feeling hungrier than normal, increase your vegetable portions by two or even three fist-sized portions. Don't worry, you won't be overeating and consuming too many calories because veggies are nutritionally dense but low in calories. I highly recommend you eat more vegetables to feel satisfied with your meals, as you can have them guilt-free.

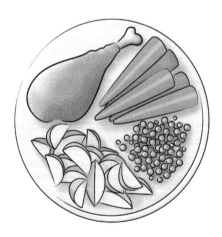

Top tip: Fruits are classed as carbohydrates, so when you eat fruit, apply the cupped hand portion. Yes, they are healthy and provide vitamins, but they do contain naturally occurring sugars too. Many fruits are high in sugar and should be eaten sparingly if your goal is to lose weight.

Food quality

Now that you know how much to eat, let's look at *what* to eat. By improving the quality of your food you will feel, look and perform at your best. This will help you get faster results in your fitness goal and is vital for long-term success.

Have you heard the saying, 'Not all calories are created equal'? The science behind it is a book in itself, but simply put, our body reacts differently to the types of food we eat. Some of these reactions are good for our health, and some (over time) are bad. The good ones keep us vital and the bad can create adverse health conditions and weight gain. Let's say we have two people who eat a diet of one thousand calories per day. Person one is Olivia: she's eating one thousand calories from a balanced, healthy diet. Person two is Alexia: she's eating one thousand calories of cheesecake every day. Essentially, the calories are the same, but the reactions (what's going on behind the scenes) are vastly different. Eating cheesecake every day produces a higher degree of weight

gain and increased risk of high cholesterol and diabetes. Alexia may also experience highs and lows in
energy throughout the day, feeling lethargic, unable
to recover from exercise, even weak from deficien-
cies. Olivia, on the other hand, is eating one thousand calories of healthy food. She's feeling energetic,
losing weight, getting in shape and recovering after
exercise. The calories are the same, but the effects are
totally different.

So, what we eat does count. Improve your food
quality by including more whole foods. These are
minimally processed foods that retain all of their
natural vitamins, minerals and other nutrients.
The term is normally applied to vegetables, fruits,
legumes and whole grains with minimal process-
ing, but it can apply to animal products too. To simplify, it's the difference between an apple and apple
pie, or steamed potatoes and crisps. The apple is a
whole food while the apple pie is not because it has
been processed and refined. There are different defi-
nitions of the 'whole-food diet': for some it must
include only organic or pesticide-free food, while
others use the same label to describe a plant-based
diet and veganism. (It's also sometimes described
as 'clean eating'.)

From my perspective, the quest for a whole-food
diet is a journey or a spectrum: it essentially comes
down to where you are starting from. If you currently eat most of your daily allowance as processed,

pre-packaged foods, fizzy drinks and so on, then the first step is to start buying more meat, grains, fruits and vegetables, swapping some of your drinks with water and cooking from scratch more often. If you're currently buying meat, grains, fruits and vegetables and cooking more often, then maybe you want to start looking at organic produce and possibly cutting down the amount of meat and animal products that you eat. It's completely up to you.

The benefits of eating whole foods include:

- Healthy weight management

- Improved mood

- Lower risk of heart disease

- Lower risk of developing diabetes

- Stronger bones

- Finding it easier to eat a balanced diet

- Improved sleep

- Improved skin

- More energy

- A longer lifespan

Let's apply this to real life. Here are a few examples of how to gradually improve your food quality by replacing it in stages.

Carbohydrates

Crackers → white bagels, breads, English muffins and wraps → whole or sprouted grain bagels, breads, English muffins and wraps.

Canned, dried, and pureed fruit with added sugar → canned, dried, and pureed, unsweetened fruit → fresh and frozen fruit.

Cereal bar → instant or flavoured oats → steel-cut, rolled or old-fashioned oats.

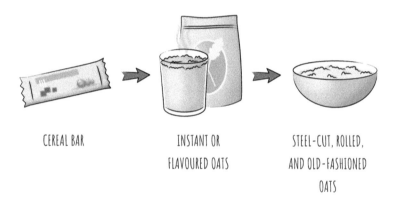

CEREAL BAR   INSTANT OR FLAVOURED OATS   STEEL-CUT, ROLLED, AND OLD-FASHIONED OATS

Protein

High-fat ground meat → medium to lean meat → lean meat (fillet beef).

Processed soy → tofu → lentils and legumes.

Fried chicken → minimally processed, lean deli meat chicken → whole fresh chicken.

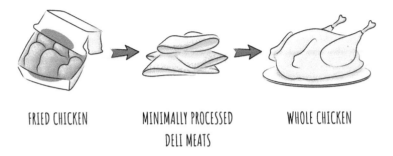

FRIED CHICKEN   MINIMALLY PROCESSED   WHOLE CHICKEN
                       DELI MEATS

Fats

Marinades and dressings → virgin olive oil → extra-virgin olive oil.

Processed cheese → cheese aged less than six months → cheese aged for six months or more.

Honey roasted peanuts → regular peanut butter → peanuts and natural peanut butter.

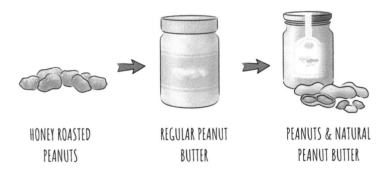

HONEY ROASTED   REGULAR PEANUT   PEANUTS & NATURAL
PEANUTS   BUTTER   PEANUT BUTTER

Vegetables

Not eating vegetables → tinned vegetables → fresh vegetables → organic vegetables.

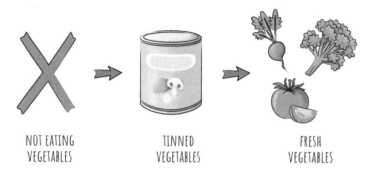

NOT EATING VEGETABLES TINNED VEGETABLES FRESH VEGETABLES

Eating whole foods means you feel fuller for longer; you feel more satisfied and your body is nourished. It also helps you to reduce your sugar intake, by reducing refined carbohydrates and sugars. This effectively promotes weight loss. For the best results, keep a close eye on your sugar consumption even from natural sources (such as fruit). The general rule is the less sugar you have, the better. Whatever your starting point, keep it simple.

Snacking

Eating whole foods also helps to reduce unnecessary snacking, and if you do snack, having the intention to improve what you eat will help you make better snack choices. It's fair to say that snacking has become an integral part of our culture. It's especially popular with Gen X and Millennials because they've grown up in a society where snacking is the norm. Many people prefer to snack simply because life is so busy that they don't have time for a proper sit-down meal. It's common to snack between meals or throughout the day, whether it's to get your energy levels up from the afternoon slump, catch a break with a snack and a drink, to comfort yourself or simply just because you're hungry.

People also choose snacks because a snack gives the impression that you're not eating much – this is common with dieters or anyone who is trying losing weight. The truth is that the average snack is packed full of calories and has little nutrition. People make the mistake of eating a snack instead of a meal because the meal looks larger, so they think they're eating more calories compared to snack food, but the reverse is often the case. Let's compare two chocolate biscuits with a bowl of ratatouille (using two fist-sized portions from the hand method). The chocolate biscuits contain 160–180 calories, with a high fat and sugar content, while the ratatouille contains 150 calories, ticks all the boxes for nutrition and promotes satiety. The meal wins. Quite often a healthy, balanced meal will outperform a snack hands down, but I know snacking can be vital for many, so my question to you is, 'What are you snacking on?'

Most people choose the tastiest options over the healthiest ones, and these are usually the high-calorie snacks packed with fats, sugars and salts. These types of snacks will certainly hold you back from getting into shape. Let's snack smartly. Snacking smartly helps to keep you satiated between meals and avoid overeating. The results of a 2016 study published in *Advances In Nutrition* showed that, 'the consumption of high-protein, high-fibre snack foods can lead to reduced caloric intake at a subsequent meal when compared with high-fat, high-sugar snack foods. Consequently, thoughtful selection of snack foods may contribute to body weight maintenance or reduction.'[10]

There are plenty of healthy snack options. These are just a few examples: apple slices with peanut butter, chia pudding, carrots with hummus, cashews with blueberries and dark chocolate, and Greek yoghurt with almonds. These types of snacks are whole foods, so they are minimally processed. Apply the food quality spectrum with snacking and ask yourself, 'How can I make this better?' If you do fancy a treat, that's fine, but begin to practise what I call 'flexible restraint'. When it comes to treats and snacks, enjoy them from time to time, but in smaller portions. Work your way up the food quality spectrum and build a diet that works for your everyday life.

---

10   V Njike et al, 'Snack food, satiety, and weight', *Advances in Nutrition,* 7/5 (2016), www.ncbi.nlm.nih.gov/pmc/articles/PMC5015032, accessed 30 March 2021

Food services

There are two common challenges that clients have expressed when implementing a healthier diet, particularly during family life. First, it's the challenge of cooking a dinner that's aligned with their wellbeing goals.

There are many reasons that you may find this difficult, for example:

- You feel tired and don't want to spend more than 20–30 minutes (if that) cooking.

- You find it hard to cook suitable meals that your children will eat too and having to cook separate meals adds to the chore.

- Your partner may not be following a healthier, calorie-reduced diet, and you may need to consider their mealtime needs, such as larger portions, including more carbohydrates in the meal, cooking meals they enjoy etc.

- You don't have enough variety in your recipe repertoire, so you get bored with your meals while trying to maintain your healthy eating routine.

The second challenge is the need to consistently eat a diet that is not only healthy but promotes weight loss. Eating to be healthy and eating to lose weight are two similar and yet different approaches. A healthy diet ('diet' used as a general term and not including specific diets) means eating a wide variety of foods from the five main food groups to get a wide range of nutrients in the right proportions. When weight loss is a consideration, not only must you eat healthily, but you must be mindful of how much you are eating, of improving your dietary habits, of maintaining a calorie deficit to promote weight loss and, most importantly, of being consistent with your diet. This requires more focus, discipline and effort.

The use of food services can simplify food preparation and help overcome lifestyle barriers to eating a healthy diet that promotes weight loss. There is a huge range of food services available, from recipe boxes to healthy readymade meals and bespoke meal plans delivered to your home. They are growing in demand and popularity because many people are increasingly health conscious but time-poor in today's fast-paced world. When clients commence their transformation plan, I suggest using food services to transition to a healthier weight loss diet easily. If dinner is the challenge, then using a recipe box service that provides healthy meals that are ready to eat in under 30 minutes is a great solution to implement, either temporarily or as an ongoing part of your new healthier lifestyle.

There are also healthy readymade meals and even bespoke meal plans, which can, for example, provide a five-day meal plan for you to follow during your busy work week and deliver your meals for the day to your home or the office. This is a great option if you don't enjoy cooking or have a busy schedule, or if you want to take the thinking process out of meal preparation.

Normally, these services are temporary but highly effective in creating good habits, helping people to eat healthier and adjust to smaller food portions. Many clients have benefited from using food services in combination with the transformation plan, and I certainly recommend you consider this when kickstarting your fitness journey.

Emotional eating

Emotional eating occurs among both genders but more commonly among women. A study asked people why they thought men and women gain weight at middle age and analysed the personal opinions of the participants. The reasons given showed that participants thought men and women in their thirties, forties and fifties gain weight for different reasons. For men, the reasons given centred on beer drinking, laziness and the fact that society is more accepting of men being overweight, so some men don't bother to get in shape. For women, on the other hand, participants in the study thought weight gain was mainly due to childbearing, hormones, menopause, sedentary lifestyle, being at home with children and comfort eating.[11]

There are many forms of emotional eating, for example, reward eating, boredom eating, loneliness eating, tiredness eating and binge eating. Comfort eating is also a form of emotional eating. We are emotional beings, and our emotions affect what we feel, think and do. There's no point in trying to fight them – they're part of who we are – but what we can do is learn to respond to them better. We can either respond to our emotions constructively or destructively.

Occasionally using food as a pick-me-up or to celebrate isn't necessarily a bad thing, but when eating is your primary emotional coping mechanism and your first impulse is to open the fridge or snack cupboard whenever you're stressed, upset, angry, lonely, exhausted or bored, you become stuck in an unhealthy cycle where the real feeling or problem is never addressed. By determining the underlying emotions that tend to drive emotional eating, it will be much easier to find a solution.

Firstly, let's differentiate between emotional hunger and physical hunger. Sometimes we can mistake the two. By identifying the signs of each, we know

---

11   S Ziebland et al, 'Body image and weight change in middle age: A qualitative study', *International Journal of Obesity*, 26 (2002), www.nature.com/articles/0802049, accessed 20 May 2021

what type of hunger we're really experiencing in that moment.

Emotional hunger	Physical hunger
Comes on suddenly	Comes on gradually
Feels like it needs to be satisfied instantly	Can be delayed
Craves specific comfort foods	Is open to various food options
Isn't satisfied with a full stomach	Stops when you're full
Triggers feelings of guilt, powerlessness and shame	Doesn't make you feel bad about yourself

Now you can recognise the signs that indicate you are eating emotionally. Maybe you didn't even know you were doing it. Different types of emotional eating demand different approaches. Realising that you have to respond to emotional hunger dependent on the circumstances is the first crucial step. I understand that addressing emotional eating can be a sensitive subject because there is an underlying reason that causes a person to emotionally eat. Not many people will address this on their own, which is why I recommend seeking a professional mentor who is able to give the appropriate guidance, support and accountability needed.

A constructive approach to overcoming emotional eating is to focus on the exact moment when you respond to your emotions with food. Before giving in to a craving, follow these steps:

Pause → recognise the situation → reflect →
decide

Most of the time, emotional eating is automatic and essentially mindless – before you even realise what you are doing there's a trail of crumbs from the pack of biscuits that's been finished. To be able to *pause*, you need something to interrupt the pattern and give you a moment to stop for a second and recognise what you are doing. This can be done by making your response foods less visible and more difficult to access. In time, this will make them unsatisfying to have, which helps to break the vicious cycle of emotional eating.

Let's use a real-life scenario: Your go-to food is sweet snacks, which are in the snack cupboard. They are all visible and easily accessible when you open the cupboard door. Start by putting all the go-to foods into a plastic bag and tying a knot so you have to physically open and close the bag. Stage two is to put the bag in a tin, so it gives you more time to pause and think about your actions when you're reaching for food as a reaction rather than hunger. If you need to, you can step it up further to stage three and put the tin in a different place where it's harder to reach and somewhat annoying to get to. How many stages you need right now depends on how often and how intensely you emotionally eat. For some, having a plastic bag and opening it up is a reminder to pause, think and decide what to do. For others, that makes no difference, so they need a more effective disruptor such as having a note attached to the bag which reads, 'Do I want to enjoy this food or am I emotionally eating?'

Clients have really benefited from this pattern of pausing, recognising the situation and deciding what to do. You will know in that moment if you're hungry or just fancy something to eat (which is fine) or if you're not feeling in a good place and responding to the situation with food. On a final note, I appreciate that for those who have children there are lots of snacks and food around the house, which is fine for them but not so great for you and your fitness goals. Without having to make it difficult to access these foods for your children, even by taking the first step of leaving a note in the cupboard can be a good start in the pause process. This creates awareness and helps to make mindful choices.

Addressing emotional eating has huge benefits – you will feel physically, emotionally and mentally better. If you are experiencing a plateau in your fitness journey this can be a breakthrough for you. If you've struggled with your weight over the years this can be a gamechanger. I'm a big advocate in overcoming emotional eating as I experienced this myself in my childhood. I've always had a good appetite and my parents liked to see me enjoy my food and finish the food on my plate. This led me to associate eating big portions with impressing my parents, receiving compliments and getting attention. In the Italian culture, the toast *salute* is commonly used and translates into 'health'. Culturally, it's not frowned upon for people to have a good appetite and to eat well, but it can be too much. I was eating like an adult at the age of ten and associated food with happiness, attention and love, and overeating became a habit. Once I began to feel unhappy with how I looked and felt and stopped caring about receiving attention from everyone, I decided it was time for change and addressed my issues. The initiative to address it and the commitment to make it happen made a huge impact and helped me to achieve my health and fitness goals.

This is intricately connected with limiting beliefs that we can carry through to adulthood. Some emotional eating can come from our childhood while other forms are developed when we are adults. When you overcome emotional eating, it's empowering and builds a new level of confidence. I experienced change, challenge and comeback in my journey, and through that experience I developed a mindset to look and feel great, not as a quick fix, but for life. I have witnessed this time and again with clients and I'm confident you can achieve it too. If this has resonated with you, try the steps mentioned in this chapter as a start and consider finding a mentor for support.

4
Move

The fourth step of the 5Ms is Move. Exercise is an important element to your overall health and a contributor to weight loss. I'm going to discuss the truth about metabolism and if we can influence it, highlight the importance of including exercise and improving your daily activity, and show you an efficient and time-saving method of exercise. I'll also share the benefits of why it's best to start exercising now rather than later.

Metabolism

I'm sure you know people who can eat anything, including junk food and never seem to gain weight. On the other hand, you probably also know people who barely eat anything and still seem to gain weight. Then there are those people somewhere in between. This raises some interesting questions about metabolism. For example, what role exactly does it play in weight gain or loss? Is our metabolic rate determined by our genes? If so, can we speed up a slow metabolism through exercise, medication or certain foods? The answer to these questions involves a mix of nature (our genetic make-up) and nurture (our environment).

Your metabolism is 'all the chemical processes that go on continuously inside your body to keep you alive and your organs functioning normally, such as breathing, repairing cells and digesting food.'[12] These require energy, and the minimum amount of energy (ie the minimum number of calories) your body requires to carry out these chemical processes is called your basal metabolic rate (BMR).

One way to think about metabolism is to view your body as a car engine that is always running. When you're sitting still or sleeping, your engine is idling like a car at a traffic light. A certain amount of energy is being burned just to keep the engine running. Of course, for humans, the fuel source is not petrol, it's the calories found in foods we eat and beverages we drink for energy. This may be used right away or stored (especially in the form of fat) for later use.

---

12 'How can I speed up my metabolism?' (NHS, October 2020), www. nhs.uk/live-well/healthy-weight/metabolism-and-weight-loss, accessed 30 March 2021

How *fast* your body's 'engine' runs on average, over time, determines how many calories you burn. If your metabolism is high (or fast), you will burn more calories at rest and during activity. A high metabolism means you'll need to take in more calories to maintain your weight – that's one reason why some people can eat more than others without gaining weight. A person with a low (or slow) metabolism will burn fewer calories at rest and during activity and has to eat less to avoid becoming overweight.

Lean people tend to be more active during every-day activities than people who are overweight. This is because they may fidget more, and they tend to be in motion even when engaged in non-exercise activities which can burn hundreds of calories each day. Although most people think it's the reverse, on average, obese people burn more calories than lean people during most activities, in part because it takes more effort to move around. They tend to be more sedentary and consume more calories than they need though, which makes it harder to get rid of body fat.

Body size, age, gender and genes all play a role in the speed of your metabolism. Muscle cells require more energy to maintain than fat cells, so people with more muscle than fat tend to have a faster metabolism. In general, men tend to have a faster metabolism because they have more muscle mass, heavier bones and less body fat than women. As we get older, we also tend to gain fat and lose muscle, which may explain why our metabolism may slow down (this accounts for both men and women).

An individual's metabolism is as specifically unique to them as their fingerprint: as far as genetics goes, we are given what we are born with. This doesn't mean someone's weight loss efforts are futile though – we don't need to rely on our metabolism, we need to focus on our lifestyle. It's part truth and part myth that metabolism is the key to weight: we cannot entirely blame excess weight on an inherited tendency to have a slow metabolism (for those who have one). Environmental factors, particularly changes in diet and exercising too little, are much more likely culprits. The reality is that for most people, excess weight is not all due to thyroid trouble, medication, bad luck, or some other unexplained, uncontrollable external factor. People who succeed in losing weight, getting in shape, and feeling better have a few things in common: they exercise regularly, reduce their calorie intake by improving their food quality and watching their food portions, and they are consistent in doing this.

It is not uncommon for people to eat more than they think they do. More often than not, the reason people put on weight isn't because of a slow metabolism, it's because they are eating and drinking more calories than they're burning. It may be hard to accept but staying on top of the number of calories you eat is key to losing weight and keeping it off. This is good news.

By improving your environment, you can achieve your health and fitness goals to look and feel great.

Regardless of whether your metabolism is fast or slow, our bodies are designed to store excess energy in fat cells, so if you eat and drink more calories (energy intake) than your body expends (energy output), you will gain weight. On the other hand, if you eat and drink fewer calories than are burned through everyday activities (including exercise, rest and sleep), you'll lose weight. Our bodies are also programmed to sense a lack of food as starvation. In response, our metabolism slows down, which means fewer calories burned over time. This is one reason why losing weight is often difficult. It's good to know that we can influence 'calories in, calories out' to determine our body size and not leave it entirely to metabolism. This means you can take positive steps to improve your lifestyle in whatever stage of life you're in now. Begin by applying Step 3 of the 5Ms to improve your diet and then add more exercise with Step 4. The combined effect will improve your quality of life and you will begin to see results.

The more you move, the better you will burn calories, and this is an essential part to lose weight, tone up and feel more energetic. Exercise has many benefits:

- It improves your sleep, mental health, mood and sexual health.

- It strengthens your bones and muscles.

- It helps keep your thinking, learning and judgment skills sharp as you age.

- It reduces your risk of heart diseases and certain cancers.

- It helps your body manage blood sugar and insulin levels.

- It reduces your risk of falls.

When you exercise, particularly exercise that makes you sweat, it generates brain-derived neurotrophic factor (BDNF), a protein which reduces stress, gets rid of cortisol (the 'fear hormone') and promotes emotional and mental wellbeing. Exercise will make you *feel* better. The following sections will show you how to move more through everyday physical activity and exercise.

Move more often

Correctly defined, physical activity is all movement that creates energy expenditure (burns calories), whereas exercise is a planned, structured physical activity such as a workout session. We live in a society where, for the most part, we are accustomed to easy accessibility and usability, time efficiency and instant results. You can order your ride on apps so you don't have to hail a taxi by the roadside; you can take a lift instead of the stairs; you can make money, have fun, research or anything you can imagine online instead of going out and playing with a ball, walking to the library or doing a physically demanding job. Global research published by the World Health Organization in 2018 found that one in three women (32%) and one in four men (23%) over the age of eighteen did not do enough physical activity and that higher-income countries have a higher prevalence of physical inactivity.[13]

In our daily lives, we are moving less. Maybe you're thinking, 'Michael, I'm running around with the kids all day long,' or, 'I'm travelling for work all the time.' I hear you. However, compare that moving around to the hours we are sedentary, whether that's sitting, commuting, working, surfing the internet on our phones or laptops (which we're likely doing sitting down), and yes, let's not forget sleeping. I am not complaining that technology has made life easier, but what is a lack of exercise doing to our health and fitness?

Exercise is indisputably one of the best natural methods for our health. If you want more energy, *get moving*, if you want to look better, *get moving*, if you want to feel less stressed, anxious or depressed, *get moving*. It's excellent for our mental, physical and emotional health and when accompanied with a healthier diet it's great for getting in shape. Diet and exercise go hand in hand

---

13 J Thornton, 'A quarter of people are not being active enough to stay healthy', *BMJ*, 362 (2018), www.bmj.com/content/362/bmj.k3796. full, accessed 30 March 2021

– it's important to combine a good diet with exercise to get the results you want to lose weight, tone up and look better. I don't prescribe exercise alone.

Does daily activity help with weight loss? This is a popular question. An analysis of the results of women between their thirties and sixties who completed their 12-week transformation plan revealed that, if you are currently sedentary, then being active every day (with or without a tailored, calorie-reduced diet) to promote weight loss is effective.

Let's start with just being active. If you are currently sedentary and not moving much during the day, then increasing your daily activity will increase your calorie burn and promote weight loss. This increase in movement is a good stimulus for your body. For the best fat-burning results, aim to be moving around every day and increasing the intensity of your daily activity. Here are ten ways to get moving more:

1. Stand rather than sit on public transport

2. Walk, cycle or run to or from work

3. Take the stairs instead of using the lift

4. Walk around during television commercials

5. Spend more time being active, eg doing household chores, DIY or gardening

6. Take walks during tea or lunch breaks

7. Set reminders to stand up every 30 minutes or so when working at a desk

8. Invest in a standing desk (or ask your workplace to provide one)

9. Find reasons to leave the office or move around the building

10. Walk around outside during phone calls

Combining this activity with a calorie-reduced diet can promote weight loss because you are creating a calorie deficit, meaning you will burn more calories than you consume. Only using daily activity to burn calories also creates a calorie deficit but the best results are a combination of exercise and diet.

You can establish how many calories you should be consuming by knowing your BMR. There are certain scales that give this info (electrical impedance scales), you can use a BMR calculator from a reputable company on the web or ask a professional to do it for you. Let us say, for example, your BMR is 1,600 calories per day. Without the need to crash-diet and dramatically dropping calories, even reducing your calories by 200–400 per day while maintaining your daily activity can be effective.

CASE STUDY: HELEN

A great example of this is when I was working with Helen. Between her work and personal commitments, she struggled to find the extra time to fit in regular exercise. She was not accustomed to doing exercise and it had never been a priority in her life, so she found it particularly challenging to motivate herself. (This is something that many people have in common so if you experience this too then don't worry, you are not alone.)

We looked to include more activity in her everyday life that would fit with her schedule. Every weekday Helen started walking 30 minutes to and from work. She gradually increased her walk to a brisk walk, followed by a power walk for the extra calorie burn and cardio benefits. In addition, we made improvements to her diet using Step 3 of the 5Ms (Meals) and within six weeks the combined effect resulted in Helen losing 3.5 kg (that's half a stone). She was absolutely delighted with the results and that was down to increasing her daily activity and a calorie-reduced eating plan specifically designed for her.

There are also long-term benefits of daily activity. Not only does moving more contribute to weight loss, but studies show that, especially for women, it is effective in preventing weight gain and maintaining a healthy weight. In a follow-up study in which the objective was to assess the relationship between physical activity and long-term weight gain, over a period of thirty-three years, women who exercised (following the recommendations given on the study) only gained 3.8 kg in that time while those who were inactive gained 9.5 kg.[14] This

---

14   C Cox, 'Role of physical activity for weight loss and weight maintenance', *Diabetes Spectrum*, 30/3 (2017), www.ncbi.nlm.nih. gov/pmc/articles/PMC5556592, accessed 30 March 2021

is equivalent to two dress sizes, which is a big difference considering losing weight can be more challenging as we get older, and a great incentive to be exercising and moving more sooner rather than later.

To get you started on the right path to looking and feeling better I want to highlight two points. First, when you start to be more active or increase your current activity, also be more mindful of how much you eat. How much we eat is connected to how much we move. When we move more, we sometimes eat more too, or we eat less when we're not exercising. One study showed that people seemed to increase their food intake after exercise either because they thought they burned off a lot of calories and could get away with eating more or because they were hungrier,[15] so when you do your exercise, be conscious of this. You also need to be careful not to overestimate how much energy your exercise has burned. You work hard exercising for 30 minutes to an hour, and that work can be erased with 5 minutes of eating afterwards. The pastry with a latte at your favourite coffee shop, for example, could undo the benefit of an hour's workout.

Some people also simply slow down after a workout, using less energy on their non-gym activities. They may decide to lie down for a rest, fidget less because

15 TS Church et al, 'Changes in weight, waist circumference and compensatory responses with different doses of exercise among sedentary, overweight postmenopausal women', *PLOS ONE*, 4/2 (2009), www.ncbi.nlm.nih.gov/pmc/articles/PMC2639700, accessed 30 March 2021

they're tired, or take the lift instead of the stairs. These changes are called 'compensatory behaviours' and refer to adjustments we may unconsciously make after working out to offset the calories burned. As a rule of thumb, keep moving on exercise and non-exercise days. Of course, it's important to listen to your body when you're feeling especially tired, but within time you will establish a good balance between rest and activity.

The second point is exercise frequency. A study showed the effects of frequency on weekly physical activity in women. The activity was walking: half the group (G1) walked for fifty minutes six times per week and the other half (G2) walked for an hour and forty minutes three times per week. Both groups followed the same prescribed dietary plan. The result? Both groups were successful in decreasing weight, body mass index and waistline, with G2 producing better results.[16] This is particularly useful for women at any age where low-impact exercise is prescribed or for older women who need low-impact exercise. The study shows that whether you do it every day or at least three times per week, you will still get results, but if you do it less frequently you do need to increase the duration of the activity. I recommend boosting your walk periodically by increasing the pace to a

---

16 A Madjd et al, 'Effect of weekly physical activity frequency on weight loss in healthy overweight and obese women attending a weight loss program: A randomized controlled trial', *The American Journal of Clinical Nutrition*, 104/5 (2016), https://academic.oup. com/ajcn/article/104/5/1202/4564398, accessed 30 March 2021

power walk for added calorie burn in less time. Over 80% of clients I worked with during their transformation plan could only exercise two to three times per week maximum. How did they achieve great results? By incorporating a holistic approach in their lifestyle which included a calorie-reduced diet with healthy food, daily activity and including HIIT as part of the two to three days of exercise.

High-intensity interval training

What if I told you that you could spend less time exercising and still see incredible results? HIIT is great for getting maximum benefits of exercise in a shorter space of time – who doesn't want that? It works by performing short bursts of intense exercise followed by less intense rest periods. A HIIT workout will typically last from 10 to 30 minutes depending on the person's fitness levels and intensity of the session.

I have found this exercise method to be a time-efficient way of burning calories, improving cardiovascular health, revving up your metabolism and seeing a significant difference in your fitness levels and body shape. I often prescribe HIIT as part of my client's exercise plan, focusing on resistance-based workouts rather than cardio alone. It is more effective to do a combination of cardio and resistance exercises together in an HIIT session than cardio alone because it maintains and builds healthy muscle, which has a metabolic effect, and our bodies burn calories more efficiently.

Here are two examples of HIIT workouts: A cardio HIIT workout would include sprinting on a treadmill for 60 seconds at +85% effort level, followed by 60 seconds walk (effort level for the rest needs to be low). Repeat these intervals 10 times. The resistance and cardio HIIT workout would include kettlebell squats, burpees, press-ups, running on the spot, kettlebell row etc, in a circuit format performing the same effort levels and timings mentioned above.

HIIT is scientifically backed to show it's an effective and time-efficient way to lose weight. A 2016 study showed that '3 minutes of intense intermittent exercise per week, within a total time commitment of 30 minutes, is as effective as 150 minutes per week of moderate-intensity continuous training'.[17] When applied correctly, HIIT works perfectly for the time-restrained individual – I have found it to be an efficient and successful exercise method.

A word of caution: HIIT may not be suitable for everyone, as it might increase the risk of injury and impose higher cardiovascular stress. This is true for individuals who are *new* to exercise, *haven't* exercised

17 JJB Gillen et al, 'Twelve weeks of sprint interval training improves indices of cardiometabolic health similar to traditional endurance training despite a five-fold lower exercise volume and time commitment', *PLOS ONE* (2016), https://journals.plos.org/plosone/article?id=10.1371/journal.pone.0154075, accessed 20 May 2021

in a long time, or may have certain *medical* conditions. Therefore, it's important to find out what your current fitness levels are and apply the appropriate plan for you. When done properly, with the correct exercises, reps/timings of each exercise and duration of the session, HIIT can be applied appropriately at most fitness levels. Without getting technical, simply put, HIIT is working hard for a set time followed by periods of less intense exercise/complete rest.

For example: If you're new to exercise, your current level of fitness might be starting with body weight squats for 45 seconds, followed by a 30–45-second rest within a circuit. Right now, that's intense for you and you're working at your near-maximum ability. This is HIIT. Soon you will progress to performing the squats at a faster pace, then adding weights, followed by doing an explosive jumping version. With all the exercises you do it's also important to listen to your body. Having muscle soreness is normal and naturally occurs a few days after a workout, but if you're feeling aches and pains in your joints, that could be a sign to reduce the intensity.

Your body adapts to exercise and so you should gradually increase the intensity of the exercise as your fitness levels and strength increase. The reality is that most people put on a fitness DVD after not exercising for months or years and start jumping around for an hour and next thing you know they've injured themselves and can't do anything. It's like telling a learner driver on their first day to start changing gears without first teaching them how to – they're bound to stall and come to a grinding halt.

Here is a safe, effective and hassle-free way of doing HIIT. I use the 'one to ten effort level' with my clients. It's a simple scale and works perfectly. Level one is easy, level five is moderate and level ten is maximum. You can judge the *intensity* of the exercise by putting an effort level to it: with HIIT, you want to aim for eight and above. The key with this method is that during the exercise phase, you need to max out your effort by performing an exercise faster, adding resistance (weights, body weight, bands, etc), choosing a more advanced exercise for your fitness levels or anything that makes it more challenging, while maintaining good form. During your rest period, focus on your breathing and getting your heart rate down to prepare for the next bout of exercise. Repeat these intervals using the effort scale of one to ten to measure the intensity of your workout. Do you remember Kathryn's success story? She benefited from HIIT and lost over 21 kg in a year by doing HIIT workouts in her sessions twice per week and played sports once per week for extra calorie burn and fun.

CASE STUDY: SARAH

I recall working with Sarah. She was in her late forties and had just had a baby. She wanted to lose her baby weight and needed guidance on how to do it safely and naturally. It's not advisable to do jumping or heavy-weighted exercises during this postnatal stage, so I applied the HIIT principle by getting Sarah to do low-impact exercises, performed at a quicker pace with strict form. As she progressed and got stronger, we gradually increased the intensity judged on how she felt and within twelve weeks Sarah had lost 7 kg (that's over a dress size). She was over the moon with her results and felt great in herself.

I'm an advocate for HIIT training and have seen great results time and again when it has been applied properly. If you have experience with exercise and you know your body well you can create or find a suitable workout plan for yourself, but if you're just getting back into exercise, haven't exercised in a while or you're not sure what to do, I highly recommend having a professional design a bespoke plan for you.

Start exercise now rather than later

Whether you're in your thirties or fifties, have just had a child or are experiencing menopause, it's never too late to start exercise. Weight loss can get harder with age, so it's better to start sooner rather than later. The reality is that not everyone will become overweight as they age. Body weight is highly influenced by your genetic make-up, your level of physical activity, and your food choices, but there is a saying that 'genetics loads the gun and lifestyle pulls the trigger'. We are going to dive into the five main contributing factors as to why you may be finding it harder to lose weight as you get older due to nature (our bodies) and nurture (our lifestyles).

You're experiencing major lifestyle changes

One of the biggest changes comes when you start a family. Before, you could spend an hour at the gym after work but now you're at home with your baby. Later, your child's after-school time is filled with playdates, homework and other activities that require your attention. You do not seem to have time for yourself anymore. As a result, your diet and exercise intentions might slip, causing a few kg to creep on. These lifestyle changes can last for a few years during the family life stage. I recommend revisiting Step 2 of the 5Ms (Motivation). Do you remember TEAM? Time, Energy, Accountability, Mentorship. If you are experiencing any or all of those challenges, they need to be resolved to successfully achieve your weight loss goals to look and feel better.

You're more sedentary and more stressed

When your career is in full swing it can pose a few weight loss and fitness challenges. For one, you are likely moving less, sitting more often and travelling for longer. You may also find yourself too busy to break for lunch, increasing the odds that you will snack on the go or order in calorie-dense takeaway food. High levels of interpersonal stress in your personal or work life can also be a contributing factor. A study found that those with high interpersonal stress had higher ghrelin and lower leptin levels than those who experienced fewer interpersonal stressors.[18] Ghrelin is the 'hunger hormone' and eating more calories over time can really add up. The same study suggests that ghrelin increases consumption of hedonically pleasant food such as food high in sugar and fat. The combination of feeling hungrier and craving junk food or fast food is a recipe for weight gain.

Stress is also linked with increased alcohol consumption, which can quickly increase your calorie intake. Enjoying certain foods and having a drink is fine, but how much and how often is the question you need to consider, especially if it's having a negative effect and you're not comfortable with how you look and feel.

Exercise helps to elevate your mood, reduce depression and release feel-good hormones which will help to destress and feel mentally and physically better. The sooner you start to exercise, the sooner you will reap the various benefits that exercise has to offer.

---

18   L Jaremka et al, 'Interpersonal stressors predict ghrelin and leptin levels in women', *Psychoneuroendocrinology*, 48 (2014), www.sciencedirect.com/science/article/abs/pii/S030645301400225X?via%3Dihub, accessed 30 March 2021

You're experiencing age-related muscle loss

The amount of lean muscle we have naturally begins to decline by 3–8% per decade after the age of thirty,[19] a process called sarcopenia. Why is this important? Because lean muscle uses more calories than fat. Unless you are regularly strength training with weights to maintain and build muscle, your body will need fewer calories each day. That makes weight gain likely if you continue to consume the same number of calories as you did when you were younger. Most people don't adjust calories, they keep eating the same amount, but because they have less muscle mass to burn those calories and are less active, they end up gaining weight over time.

Include more resistance exercise into your fitness routine, aiming for a minimum of twice per week. To reduce age-related muscle loss, also keep an eye on protein. Most people tend to eat the lower end of their daily requirement for protein, so aim to include a variety of plant-based and animal-based protein in each meal and snacks.

Your metabolism is slower than before

The decrease in muscle mass is likely to slow your metabolism, a complex process that converts calories

---

19   E Volpi et al, 'Muscle tissue changes with aging', *Current Opinion in Clinical Nutrition and Metabolic Care*, 7/4 (2010), www.ncbi.nlm.nih. gov/pmc/articles/PMC2804956, accessed 30 March 2021

into energy. Having more fat and less muscle reduces calorie burning, and as mentioned earlier, you're less active with age, so your body is burning calories less efficiently.

You're undergoing normal hormonal changes

Both men and women undergo changes in hormone levels as part of aging, which helps to explain why middle age is prime time for putting on pounds. For women, menopause (which occurs most often between ages forty-five and fifty-five) causes a significant drop in oestrogen. This encourages extra weight to settle around the stomach. The shift in fat storage may make the weight gain more noticeable and increase health-related risks.

In addition, fluctuations in oestrogen levels during perimenopause, the years leading up to menopause, may cause fluctuations in mood that make it more difficult to stick to a healthy diet and exercise plan. A study showed that the average weight gain during the transition to menopause is about two to four kg.[20] This phase can create a snowball effect: you start accumulating more fat, you have less lean body mass, you burn less calories and this just keeps adding up over time.

---

20 G Panotopoulos et al, 'Weight gain at the time of menopause', *Human Reproduction*, 12 (1997), https://doi.org/10.1093/humrep/12.suppl_1.126, accessed 30 March 2021

The solution

Start exercising, do it frequently and stick with it. Remember the golden rule: *keep it simple.* That's easier said than done, isn't it? So, let's start this together. Don't wait for tomorrow, or next week or when you come back from holiday, but today. Take a few minutes to write down any activity or exercise that you can start with the least amount of resistance. Begin by answering the following questions:

- Am I motivated to exercise alone, do I prefer a group environment, or do I need that extra push with one-to-one mentorship?

- What will be the easiest option to get me started? (The key to starting and maintaining exercise is having minimal barriers, because it requires less motivation on your part and fewer excuses/reasons to not do it.)

- How much time do I have?

- Do I have time to commute to my exercise venue?

- Will commuting be a barrier? (Often getting there is half the battle.)

- How much time do I have in my current schedule – is it 10 minutes, 30 minutes or 1 hour?

- How often can I realistically fit in weekly exercise?

Now give some thought as to what you enjoy doing. For example, do you enjoy:

- Playing a sport

- Exercise classes

- Dance classes

- Home exercising with a DVD

- One-to-one personal training

- Going to the gym

- Walking every day for 30 minutes

- A combination of the above

Answering these questions will give you clarity. Whatever you choose, you will benefit from exercising sooner rather than later. If you need that extra push and support, use the TEAM approach to guide you.

5
Maximise

We have looked at Mindset, Motivation, Meals and Move. The final stage of the 5Ms is Maximise. In this step, you will learn to recognise the difference between success and failure in achieving your goals, why it's important to focus on your behaviours (what you do), how habits can help you can stay in shape for a lifetime, and the secret ingredient to seeing lasting results: consistency.

Time for action

Firstly, let's look at taking action. Most people get stuck when it comes to *doing* something about their goals. This is the point at which you either succeed or fail. You may experience some ups and downs in your fitness journey but remember that this is normal and OK. When do you remember anything worth achieving being plain sailing? Those down moments are not failures – they're learning curves and a part of the experience. Failure is not trying at all; failure is the story we tell ourselves to prevent any mistakes from happening or to avoid challenges. Failure is to avoid confronting the fear that stops us from starting anything in the first place, or which stops us from persevering with what we want to accomplish.

If you are telling yourself that you want to look and feel great and it brings a smile to your face when you envision yourself in the future having more energy, feeling stronger, fitter and looking amazing in your clothes, then it's time to maximise to make that a reality. The fact that you're reading this means you've invested time and effort in learning how to become a better version of yourself for your mind, your body and your health. You're now equipped with everything you need to get started and my advice to you is to start your fitness journey asap.

The 5Ms will work when you do them at your own pace, whether that means one step at a time such as focusing on your diet first and then moving on to exercise, or full steam ahead and applying everything in one go. If you start and follow the steps of each stage in order, there is no right or wrong. Personally, I'm an all-or-nothing kinda guy. I throw myself into the zone and I figure it out as I go along, but I've learned from coaching clients that we all have different ways of doing things.

You should approach your fitness routine in a way that works for you. Most people are either step-by-step or all-or-nothing personalities. You will know which type of person you are. If you go all-or-nothing into your fitness routine but you're a step-by-step person, you will soon feel overwhelmed, stressed and unhappy. On the other hand, if you're an all-or-nothing person but you approach it step by step, you will lose interest, become impatient, give up the whole fitness routine entirely and probably feel crap for not accomplishing it.

Here's an example of where to start if you are a step-by-step person: make one improvement in your diet such as reducing your portion sizes. Only focus on that without changing the way you eat, that will come next, but give yourself some time to adjust with the portions first. Start by reducing your portions at dinner and once you are accustomed to that (usually a few days) move on to improving your lunch portions, followed by breakfast. This is less overwhelming and gives you time to adjust and stick to it long term. Once you've accomplished this, move on to improve what you eat and begin including exercise in your routine.

Start increasing your physical activity by walking more with intervals of jogging throughout your walk twice per week. After a few weeks, increase the exercise to three times per week and commit to that for a while. As you get into a routine with your fitness plan, you can improve your diet and exercise as you go along and step it up to the next level. Now that you have an idea of how to start and make it part of your new lifestyle, go for it. I'm cheering you on.

All-or-nothing people, here we go: you're ready to go all in and likely to be starting exercise and making changes to your diet at the same time, so it's best to plan and prepare – creating automation will be your route to success. Schedule exercise in your diary on a recurring basis. If it changes, then set a reminder in your calendar or an alarm to schedule in your exercise sessions for the week ahead. Do the same with your food shopping (if you shop online, create a 'saved' basket of your favourite items, this is a supremely time-efficient way of doing it). Follow Step 3 of the 5Ms (Meals) by improving your quality of food, and putting your favourite healthy choices in your weekly shopping basket or choosing a healthy food service.

All-or-nothing people are more likely to eat and drink whatever they want and when they want, which is why they're more prone to gaining weight when they're not eating right. On the flip side, they follow a healthier eating plan rigorously and stick to it, which helps them to lose a good amount of weight in a good timeframe. My advice is to apply the hand portions approach straight away and improve the quality of your current weekly food shop with as many items as you can. There will be a time when you step out of the small 'circle' and it's the all-or-nothing people who generally struggle the most here, because if you're going to drink, you're not just going to have a glass – you may have the entire bottle. For you to successfully see a difference in your body shape, drop a dress size or more, and feel better, going back to this approach will not work.

It's the mindset of having in excess that makes all-or-nothing people yo-yo with their weight: you look and feel amazing for months because you've been great with your diet and exercise, but when you're in the opposite direction it all comes back on and the good habits fly out the window.

CASE STUDY: LAURA

Laura is a mum of three and has a busy corporate job and an active social life. She found it hard to lose weight because chocolate and alcohol were her Achilles heel and when she did have them, she went all out. She found it incredibly hard to change her mindset. During her transformation plan Laura didn't lose any weight in the first six weeks and felt disheartened because she was taking one step forward and two steps back due to her food intake. I suggested that she avoid her Achilles heel (no chocolate or alcohol) for just one week, and in that week she lost 2 kg. It may not sound like much, but for her it was a breakthrough after years of not being able to lose weight.

Laura was so delighted with the result that it sparked the motivation to persist with her plan and put more effort into her approach. This led to her achieving her goal of losing two dress sizes. She was ecstatic, and the best part was that when Laura reintroduced chocolate and alcohol into her life, she didn't have it in excess like she used to. She felt great and didn't want to ruin that feeling. Laura needed time to rewire her mindset, attitude and habits to develop a new, healthier and balanced relationship with food, but she couldn't have done it without deciding to stop her all-or-nothing behaviours.

I'm pleased to say that Laura continues to exercise regularly, eats healthily and whenever she does want to eat something outside of the 'circle' she does it guilt-free now that she has found balance. Embracing balance doesn't happen overnight, but by starting now you can look and feel great over a lifetime rather than sometimes.

Focus on your behaviours as much as your goals

Behaviours are what you do, so focusing on them means to mindfully make the best possible choices, act based on those choices and be consistent with your actions (what you are doing). A goal is the object of a person's ambition or a desired result. It is good to have a goal because it provides clarity on what you want and when you want it. To achieve effective weight loss results, it is important to focus on your behaviours as much as your goals.

Let's use this scenario to understand why focusing on your behaviour is the route to success: Miranda's goal is to lose 10 kg in six months. She regularly weighs herself to see if she's lost weight. The only thing that's important for her is seeing the numbers go down to achieve her goal. When they do go down, she's happy and feels great and this motivates her to keep making good decisions as part of her lifestyle. When the numbers go up or stall, she's demotivated and gives up her good efforts by falling back into bad habits and making poor choices that don't contribute to her well-being goals.

One of the reasons why most people struggle to lose weight and don't achieve their goal of looking and feeling better is because they weigh themselves too often and allow the weight scales to dictate their actions. This is common if someone has just started a fitness plan or has a weight loss goal, it's understandable, you want to check that what you are doing is correct and to see that all your hard effort is paying off. Like Miranda, most people focus only on the numbers going down to achieve their goals. Miranda's behaviours are based on the up and down results on the scale, and it's here that people can either take a long time to achieve their desired outcome or never achieve it, because eventually they give up.

Humans are emotional beings, and when we focus on our health and fitness goals there is an emotional component. This is why the weight scale has so much influence on our behaviours, because more often than not we process the result with our emotions rather than with rational thinking. It's the way we are wired. In Miranda's scenario, she weighs herself every other day. When the scales show she's losing weight, she feels slim but when the weight is up, she feels fat, even though it's only been a day. Sound familiar? A study in Poland showed that women 'with higher body mass and longer waist circumferences had a higher level of negative body perception, but no similar significant correlation was found in men.'[21] The important part of this study is that 67% of the women were a healthy weight (neither overweight nor obese) and yet their perceptions of themselves were negative. A separate study examining body image and personal happiness revealed that 'happiness significantly and positively correlated with the three components of body esteem: sexual attractiveness, weight concern and physical condition.'[22] In a scenario like Miranda's, imagine the effect that weighing yourself every day and getting mixed messages will have on what you think about yourself?

---

21 A Demuth et al, 'Subjective assessment of body image by middle-aged men and women', *Studies in Physical Culture and Tourism*, 19/1 (2012), www.wbc.poznan.pl/Content/217190/PDF/8_Demuth_25_29.pdf, accessed 30 March 2021

22 R Stokes et al, 'Women's perceived body image: Relations with personal happiness', *Journal of Women and Aging* (2008), www.tandfonline.com/doi/abs/10.1300/J074v15n01_03, accessed 30 March 2021

Focusing on your actions and progress by consistently making the best possible choices with your food, exercise, sleep, stress levels and overall lifestyle and giving yourself credit for doing so will help you achieve your goals, and better enjoy the process.

CASE STUDY: KAREN

Karen has two children and works for a FTSE 100 company. Her goal was to lose two dress sizes, but she struggled to find the time and energy to commit to a fitness routine on her own. Her work was stressful and demanding, and her home life, although less stressful, left her with little time to focus on herself.

To begin with, Karen adhered to her transformation plan, but even with the support of a coach, she still lacked the motivation to make good choices throughout the day. When we talked about her routine, she told me that she was weighing herself every day. Now it all made sense. When she stepped on the scale and the results were good, she was happy and her good actions continued for the day, but when it was the opposite, she felt upset and frustrated, and regressed to bad habits. When Karen weighed herself every day, it created a mindset which affected her decision-making based on how she felt.

On the good days, if Karen fancied chocolate, she followed the hand portions and would choose dark chocolate over milk or white chocolate because it was in alignment with her new, healthier diet. On the bad days, because she was upset, she ate the whole bar. Even with her exercise, on good days Karen would do her own workouts outside of our sessions, but on bad days she couldn't be bothered and found any excuse not to do it because she'd lost her motivation from the morning's results on the scales.

Karen was in a behavioural pattern of taking one step forwards and two steps back, so she stopped weighing herself and committed to our scheduled fortnightly tracking. This made a world of a difference. Within a few weeks she'd lost 2 inches off her waist. Why? Karen did all her exercise, followed the eating routine and stuck with it. She was so happy with the results and amazed that she had been self-sabotaging without being aware of it.

Karen continued to focus on her actions which set her up for success the next day, the next week and the next month to lose her desired weight. She achieved her goal of losing two dress sizes in less than six months by focusing on her behaviours and following the 5Ms.

Tracking progress

To help you focus on your actions, I'm going share with you how often you should weigh yourself, different ways of tracking your progress to continually lose weight, and why this method works.

Start by committing to weighing yourself once every two weeks – weight gain or weight loss is a process, it takes time for your body to either lose or gain weight. It's normal for our body weight to change daily because of many factors such as water and food intake, water retention due to sodium and carbohy-drates, excretion of urine and stool and other factors like medication, alcohol intake and menstrual cycles in women. With so many variables, stepping on the scales too often will not give a true picture of whether you've lost weight.

Two weeks also allows enough time to focus on micro-goals. These are small goals you give yourself on a daily or weekly basis, such as, 'This week I'm going to reduce my alcohol to one glass instead of two or three,' or, 'I'm going to increase my exercise to two workouts instead of one.' These small goals contrib-ute to the effectiveness of your weight loss and are manageable because you only need to focus on two weeks at a time for when you do your fortnightly check-ins. If the results are not showing after two consecutive weigh-ins, then this is a good indicator that further improvements in your lifestyle need to be made (a good reason to track your progress to give you feedback on what you are doing).

Secondly, measure your progress in different ways, don't just stick with one. There are four ways to track your progress: body measurements, using your clothes, a weight scale and visually.

Body measurements

This is on the top of my list and my clients' favourite too. Why? People store fat in different places of the body and there is usually a specific area that never seems to budge. For some it might be the stomach and for others it's on the side of the hips – whichever it is, it's the hardest to get rid of, but also the most satisfying to achieve when you see improvement in that area. Measurements are a more reliable progress indicator than weight scales and also a great way to see how your body shape is changing and where you're toning up.

Using your clothes

People lose weight for various reasons, and if yours is to look and feel better, what better way to measure your progress than how you look in your clothes? It's a great feeling when you fit into favourite clothes that you haven't worn for a while because they were too tight or felt uncomfortable. As you progress with your goals you might even need a new wardrobe – if you love shopping this gives you a perfect excuse.

Weight scales

It's better to have a scale that reads more than just weight. Insights such as your body fat percentage, muscle mass and BMR will give you a bigger picture of your body's composition. A lot of people focus only on the scales and don't try the other measurements, but I encourage you to do all four factors to keep you on track with your fitness plan.

Visual improvements

You will get natural feedback when you look at yourself in the mirror. Over time, you will notice improvements in various areas of your body. This is a great motivational and confidence booster.

Take the high-speed train to looking and feeling great by being consistent with what you do, tracking your progress using the four methods and celebrating little triumphs.

Habits

Habit derives from the Latin word *habere*, which means 'to hold' and 'to keep'. Its English definition is 'an action performed repeatedly and automatically, usually without awareness'. It's good to understand the origin because habits are actions that we keep, often for our entire lives, and they can affect us both positively and negatively.

From a health and fitness perspective, you want to form habits that will positively influence your goals while reducing and even eliminating habits that inhibit you from achieving your goals. Habits will not only aid with results but will also make them last. Clients who continue to look and feel great long after completing their transformation plan have their habits to thank. I'm no longer there to keep them accountable, provide guidance and support to ensure they stay committed; it's now down to them. During the process of the transformation plan they have created habits that positively influence their lifestyle and are now part of their lives. Forming habits is a process – on average, it takes three months to form a habit. The more meaningful our *why*, the faster we embrace and implement these habits.

New habits are formed by having a conscious reason to form them. This is done by knowing how you will benefit from this new habit, for example, forming a new habit to eat less snack food or drink less alcohol late at night while watching television, as this will improve your quality of sleep to feel more rested and energised the next day. This new habit will contribute to achieving your goal of losing 10 kg in six months because the more energy you have, the better your level of motivation to adhere to your fitness routine.

Here's a top tip from a perfectionist veteran for the perfectionists out there: put your perfectionism to one side. Successfully creating habits is about being prolific, not perfect. Perfectionism can bring your fitness triumphs to a halt. Being prolific is to 'start, improve and continue what you do'. It's acting and improving the quality of what you're doing along the way. For example, when you start exercising it might just be 10 minutes of jogging once a week. You can then improve it by increasing to fifteen to 20 minutes of jogging twice a week and continue to do so until you have built yourself a good exercise routine that you can maintain.

Perfectionism means refusal to accept any standard short of perfection, which for your fitness routine translates into rigorous, strict and unattainable in everyday life. You need to allow some flexibility – it's called balance. Having a good balance will give you the mind space to make changes in your food, exercise and lifestyle and stick to it without feeling stressed and overwhelmed. You will have the accountability needed to form habits without the additional pressure.

It is also important to celebrate your triumphs in your fitness journey as this will encourage your good habits and reduce negative ones. Take a moment to celebrate your accomplishments, no matter how big or small. This will encourage you, give you more confidence and make your fitness journey easier and fun. Learn to support, affirm and be proud of yourself, rather than be critical. The worst disservice you can do to yourself is to undercut your successes. This type of negative thinking is more harmful than helpful since it devalues your efforts. What happens if you do that? All the good actions you're doing and the habits you're forming go flying out the window. The size of the celebration doesn't matter – it's the recognition. Think about a time when someone complimented you: how great did it feel? We must learn to also do this for ourselves: recognise all the good behaviours we're doing and feel good about them. When you're tracking your progress and have lost an inch here and there, that's a step forward. Tell someone who is supportive in your fitness journey and celebrate it. By doing this, it is easier to be consistent with your new healthy habits.

To stay consistent with your habits, also avoid the trap of comparing yourself to others. I've seen this before with clients and it can derail a person in their efforts to achieve their goals. Each person is at a different place in their lives and fitness journeys. It is self-defeating to believe you must be successful or be healthy in a fixed amount of time. Focus on your journey and follow the 5Ms until you reach your goal of living a healthier and happier life. Remember, everyone is on a different journey but with the same result: to look good and feel great about themselves. To form new habits, you need to have a reason to do so, remind yourself throughout your fitness journey of the benefits of this new habit and give yourself credit for doing it and sticking with it.

Consistency is success

The effectiveness of consistency is understated in the fitness world. There's always a lot of hype about a new exercise or diet or a trendy new fitness movement, which is fine – everything has its place. What doesn't get promoted is the importance of being consistent in achieving your health and fitness goals.

I guess picking up a magazine with a headline that reads 'The No 1 Secret to Losing Weight is Consistency,' doesn't sound attractive compared to 'Do These 10 Fat-burning Exercises for a Flatter Tummy'. The truth is that weight loss doesn't need to be complicated. The journey can be challenging at times, but the process doesn't need to be. It's consistency in following all of the 5Ms – Mindset, Motivation, Meals, Move and Maximise – to the best of your ability that will pay off. It really is as simple as that.

The truth is that most people don't succeed in looking and feeling better because they are inconsistent. They either have a reason or an excuse, and while some are well-founded and unavoidable, the good news is there are generally solutions for most obstacles. Here are a few common, real-life scenarios of why people find it hard to be consistent with their exercise, food, and lifestyle choices and some guidance on how to overcome them.

You're not seeing changes in your body

Everyone likes instant results, who doesn't? I do. Some things can be achieved instantly but others take a bit of time. I don't know how big or small your goal is, but on average it can take up to twelve weeks of a fitness routine to see noticeable changes. That's why the transformation plan is twelve weeks, because you need that time to apply everything consistently and the results will show. Now, you might be thinking,

'But Michael, I did all the right things. I improved my diet. I'm exercising more and even sleep better now. Why haven't I seen any change?' The reality is people lose weight at different paces. For some, it will take longer to lose weight or see any results. Others lose weight at a steady pace, they will track their results every week or so and they will hit their target goal consistently, give or take. Others respond immediately to a fitness plan and get incredible results in a short space of time.

There are many variables that contribute to how quickly you will see results, but here are three things to consider in assisting you to set realistic goals and have an idea of how long it will take you to achieve them:

- **Importance:** The first on the list is how important or significant something is because I've learned from my actions, my client's actions and studying people in general that when something is important to us, humans are incredible at making the impossible possible. The point I'm making is that if your fitness goals are truly meaningful to you, you will find the time, you will make the effort and you will find the resources to achieve your goal of looking and feeling great.

- **Time:** If you compare a twenty-year-old college student who has time on her hands and fewer responsibilities to a forty-year-old woman who has children and is working, the timeframe and method of achieving their results is understandably different. The college student can train five times per week and get solid sleep for recovery while the working mother of two will sleep less and can only fit in two, maybe three workouts a week at a push (this is often more challenging for single parents who don't have the additional support network from their partners). The better you manage and prioritise time for yourself, the better the results, because you will have a good weekly momentum. Your time is not just for your exercise, but also to plan food shopping for the week ahead, cook healthy meals, give yourself more downtime to reduce stress, or have more rest to recover mentally and physically.

- **Resources:** Everyone has a different budget, and this will affect the quality of food you buy, such as basic brand or organic, and the fitness services you choose, whether you choose to run (which is free for anyone), go to a gym or hire a personal coach.

Each of these factors will dictate the pace at which you will see results to some extent. If you're not seeing changes in your body, go through the 5Ms and see if there's anything missing in your fitness routine.

You don't enjoy exercise

Find a routine that fits your personality and lifestyle. If you're new to exercise then it may feel difficult at the start, and that's normal, but once you get fitter and stronger it gets better. If you're struggling to commit to a specific routine, then maybe it's not the right one for you. There is more to exercise than just going to the gym: you can choose from a variety of options such as group fitness, working out at home, using a fitness app, using exercise DVDs, playing a sport, exercising outdoor in nature or having one-to-one coaching – the choice is yours.

You keep quitting

You might start out strong and with the best intentions, but before you know it, you've lost your motivation. People quit because of four possible reasons:

- **They do too much too soon:** If you go from no exercise at all to exercising seven days a week, eventually you're bound to feel burned out. Instead, ease into a new routine.

- **Confusion:** If you're confused with what to do with your diet and exercise, two options are do your research to find out what's best for you or hire a professional to do it for you. This will give you clarity and keep you motivated.

- **Boredom:** Anything monotonous will fail sooner or later. We all need new stimuli and variety, but at the same time we also need certainty that doing the right things will deliver great results. Add variety to your exercise routine by choosing a few activities from those listed earlier. Try new ingredients and recipes and use food services that suit you. I insist that my clients add variety to their fitness routines because they will enjoy it more and that means being consistent.

- **Soreness:** When you're just starting out, soreness is to be expected, but you should still be able to function. If you're so exhausted after your workout that you can't lift your head off the pillow or you get an injury while exercising, you're not likely to feel motivated to get back to it once you're feeling better. I mentioned the effort level scale of one to ten in the HIIT chapter – use that to determine the intensity of an exercise and adjust it to your fitness levels accordingly.

You can't commit

When you only think about exercise in the long term (I must do this *forever*), it can be overwhelming. You don't have to change everything in your life all at once, and not all the changes you make must happen overnight. If you're having trouble sticking to your workout routine, go back to your *why* and try to make exercise a priority. Ask yourself if a fitness routine is important to you or if you just want it to be. Making exercise a priority takes commitment, and commitment takes motivation. Your *why* will power you through and give you the motivation to be consistent. Start with small goals and plan to make them achievable, it's easier to stick with a workout when your goals start small. Try including more daily activity and challenge yourself to walk an extra 10 minutes each day. From there you can progress to including a workout session every week, and so on.

If your only goal is weight loss, don't focus just on that. It can be difficult to stick to a routine if you don't see results right away. While you don't want to lose sight of your long-term goals, try to focus on the other benefits of exercise and eating healthier such as the positive feeling you get for living this way. Commitment can be successfully achieved by having a routine in place. Following the TEAM section in Step 2 of the 5Ms will help you to create a routine.

You don't know how to exercise

Being an exercise beginner can be overwhelming (and even intimidating). In fact, in a survey found that one of the biggest factors determining whether a person would go to the gym was confidence, particularly how confident they felt while in the gym.[23] There are many different types of exercise you can try. Some will work for you and others might not. Figuring that out for yourself can be challenging. The good news is that there are plenty of resources out there to help. If you prefer a safe and effective approach, it's best to work one-to-one with a coach to start with, move on to group exercise, and then work on your own with the knowledge and experience you've gained.

---

23 'Top excuses people use for not going to the gym' (Better, no date), www.better.org.uk/content_pages/top-gym-excuses, accessed 20 May 2021

You're too stressed

Being stressed can make everything more difficult to face. Having accountability from your support network will make it a whole lot easier to achieve your goals. If you're currently feeling stressed, exercise and a balanced diet will be beneficial for your mind and body. If this sounds overwhelming or too difficult then you will greatly benefit from having someone to hold you accountable and to set you up for success.

You have childcare responsibilities

With school and after-school activities, kids and teens can have schedules as busy as their parents. Just because you have carpool duty or need to make sure your teen gets to practice on time doesn't mean you have to neglect your own fitness goals. In fact, exercise can be a great activity for the whole family. Making time for a workout doesn't just benefit your health, it also sets a good example for your kids. Try including them into your fitness routine – yes, it will require some planning, but it's not impossible. The section about focusing on yourself in Step 1 of the 5Ms (Mindset) will also help you to prioritise your time.

You don't have time

When you're looking at your to-do list, it might feel like you just don't have time to exercise or cook a separate meal for yourself, but exercise doesn't need to take up a lot of time to be effective. Introduce the HIIT method into your routine for time-saving workouts. With food, improve your portions and food quality step by step. This will potentially benefit the whole family – I can't promise your kids will be eating a variety of rainbow-coloured veggies, but they will be encouraged to try. The key is repetition, repetition, repetition.

Those are some of the most common scenarios people experience. We all have our own reasons or excuses at some stage or another and it's reassuring to know that we're not alone. I had my own when I was a teenager, all my clients have had their own reasons or excuses, and now they have their own success stories. It is possible to become the best version of yourself.

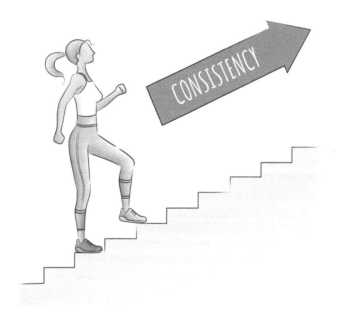

The 80/20 rule

I would like to introduce to you a concept which over the years has been incredibly successful in keeping people committed and consistent with their health and fitness routines. It's called the '80/20 rule'. What most people want to do is chill out and watch their favourite TV series with the hope of burning calories and losing weight or not having to get up 30 minutes earlier to fit in their workout. Most people want to eat what they want, whenever they want (and let's be honest, what we want generally isn't low in sugar, salt, fat and carbs) and stay slim and healthy for the rest of their lives. That's what people *want* to do, and it sounds ideal – who doesn't want to do all that most of time while looking and feeling amazing? What we *have* to do for the majority of the time to achieve our health and fitness goals is the opposite. We need to do a morning workout; eat wholesome, healthy food; be consistent every week, etc. This doesn't mean we can't do both: we just need to discover the balance between want and have so that we can simultaneously enjoy life and achieve our goals to lose weight, feel better and have more energy.

How does the 80/20 rule help with exercise and food adherence? Allowing yourself to do what you want 20% of the time keeps you accountable to do what you have to do 80% of the time. If you are at all like my clients or you're not being paid to be 100% consistent and committed (eg bodybuilders, models, social media influencers), then this is a way to stay motivated in your fitness routine and have the freedom to enjoy life. If you like what you're hearing by not being tied down to regimental diet plans and extreme exercise and having a routine that fits in your lifestyle for a lifetime then I recommend that you give this concept a go. If you're sceptical, let me ask you this about previous diet plans: How long did you adhere to them? Did they get in the way of your social life? Could you have done them for a lifetime?

If you've got positive answers for all three of those questions and you're happy with how you look and feel, I'm genuinely pleased for you because you have found a diet that works for you, fits into your life and allows you to live in optimal health. If not, it's highly likely it's another 'diet plan' that's simply not attainable and I urge you try the 80/20 rule to help you be consistent in following the 5Ms. What I want for you more than anything is for you to achieve your goals and live the best version of yourself for as long as you can, I dare to say a lifetime. It may sound unattainable, but it really is possible, because lifestyle means the way in which a person lives. Having a balance such as the 80/20 rule creates consistency, consistency connects with habits and habits are your *lifestyle*. They coexist.

I recall working with Sophie. She had an extremely busy social life, so there was a lot of drinking and eating involved, and she knew that this wasn't going to change any time soon. I suggested applying the 80/20 rule. Every week, Sophie needed to follow her exercise routine and diet for 80% of the time. The 20% covered times when she had a social event and wanted to have an extra glass of wine with friends or unexpected, real-life events such as running late after a meeting and being too tired to cook, so snacking on something instead. This only works when you draw a line under that 20%, because if that glass becomes three or four, you're no longer on track, or if you consistently come home late but don't have the right food ready, you won't see results.

With my clients, I record everything they communicate with me to track their progress and keep them in the balance of 80/20. I'm not saying this is what you have to do, but when you reflect on your week, ask yourself how you've scored out of ten (ten equals excellent and one equals terrible). For example, you did your exercise, you managed stress better and followed your improved diet for every meal, while enjoying a Wednesday dinner with friends and a Saturday lunch with the family – you can honestly rate yourself eight. Remember, your score doesn't need to be perfect, but to see results and lose weight it does need to be very good.

Simple and powerful... but will you succeed?

What I have shared with you may seem simple. I've given you five areas to focus on. You'll start to see this formula everywhere now that you know it. Friends, family, colleagues – anyone in your social circle that has achieved impressive weight loss results has followed the 5Ms with or without knowing it. Built into these five outcomes of becoming the best version of yourself, you will find that there is confidence, strength, vitality and joy. Over the next few months, I can guarantee you that there will be new success stories of clients who have completed their 12-week transformation plans and achieved incredible results. My inbox will be full of women who have read this book and shared their success stories of following the method. I know what they will say. Their emails will tell me that they put in the effort, pushed through their limiting beliefs, made the time, and did all five steps in order (it's important that the five steps are done in order). They will tell me that, as I promised, they have a healthier lifestyle, they are happier, they look better and feel good within themselves.

I sincerely want you to be one of those success stories. I want your story in my inbox saying that you have done these five simple things, you've lost weight, you have more energy, you're living a healthier life and you're feeling good about yourself. Sadly, there's a good chance you won't be. People can get caught up in the struggle and let complexity get in the way of simplicity. People cut corners for the desire of immediate quick wins or give up before they've achieved their full potential and seen results. Over the last ten years, working with women who are busy, hardworking mothers, I've analysed decision-making habits. As a body transformation coach, it's my responsibility to understand human behaviour and its influence on how people make decisions and take action for wellbeing goals in their life. In the final chapter I will share some of the things I have noticed when watching people with similar challenges and goals successfully achieve them or perpetually get stuck. I will offer some ideas on how you can overcome these obstacles to look and feel great and live a healthier and happier life.

6
Make It Happen

If you've made a decision, then you need to act on it. Whatever stage of life you're in right now, you have the blueprint to look and feel great. It's time to start your fitness journey.

Implementing the 5Ms

I think many of us are particularly good at making things complicated. We don't mean to, but quite often we think, 'Surely it can't be that simple? If it were, everybody would be doing it.' The reality is that with many things in life the methodology *is* simple – it's the execution of the methodology that is the challenging part. We can create complexity by focusing on the wrong things, being side-tracked during the process, cutting corners to get immediate results (what we really want is instant gratification), striving for perfectionism and self-sabotage.

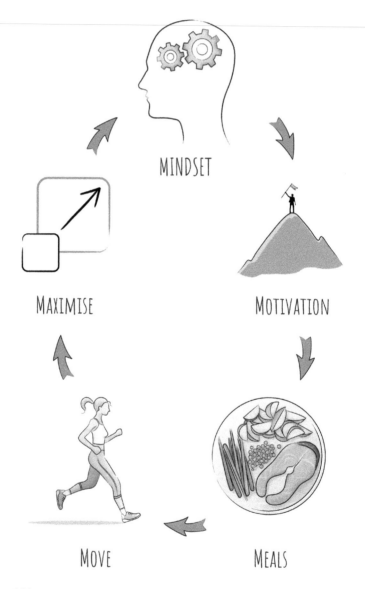

Begin with asking yourself your *why*. This is so important, because it is this answer that gives purposeful meaning to your decision-making. From there, follow it through with breaking down barriers using Step 2 (Meals). The complexity starts with the barriers which create reasons or excuses for not being able to achieve your outcome. If a barrier is other than one of those mentioned in the book, for example, an underlying health condition, a physical disability, specific hormonal imbalances or anything specific that is affecting you, consult with the appropriate professionals to give you the best advice. This will help create realistic expectations of your wellbeing goals.

From there, follow through the remaining steps one at a time, using this book as a guide. Remember, if you feel you can't do this alone, that's fine – in fact, those who achieve amazing results often have a small team behind them. My clients have me to achieve their goal of 'losing weight, getting in shape and having more energy' and quite a few of them also use physiotherapists, masseuses, GPs, specialists and food service providers to maintain a good bill of health and further aid in achieving their goals, just as you and I use multiple services for different areas of our lives.

Overcoming obstacles

At the start of my fitness career, I worked for a global gym company in London. Before you began working with them you had to do a three-day training course to familiarise yourself with the company culture, learn the ropes and, more importantly, understand their members. The company shared statistics identifying three specific member types, which I found shocking at the time but that came as no surprise once I knew the cause behind them. Their stats showed that only 5% of members attended the gym four times a week or more. These were the sportspeople and fitness buffs that knew exactly what they were doing and got on with their own fitness routine. Next, it showed that 20% of members attended once or twice a week and did a combination of classes, their own gym workout and were happy to receive some guidance from fitness instructors. Finally, the largest proportion of members, making up 75%, were members who attended the gym regularly for the first three months of joining. After that time, they either stopped or would sporadically attend throughout the year, but without a routine or any real intention. I'm certain they had a purpose, but little intention to go with it. The company gave us these statistics to help improve the member retention rate, but the reason I'm sharing this is to show you why 75% of members in a gym company that had over one million members did not achieve their health and fitness goals.

Have you connected the dots? It's because of not overcoming the TEAM obstacles: Time, Energy, Accountability, Mentorship. The members were a broad demographic consisting of men and women ranging in age from eighteen through to their eighties, each with varied goals and their own journeys. However, the statistics show that we essentially all pretty much experience the same challenges. We all have twenty-four hours in a day – it's down to us how we spend it. Energy equals output, and if our energy (mental or physical or both) is affected, it has a knock-on effect on output. Accountability is needed, by our own means or from motivation and support from others. Finally, a mentor can show us what to do, how and when do it, and guide and support us along the journey. Sometimes it can feel that the only person who experiences the struggles and challenges is you, but we all experience them. The 5Ms breaks through those challenges to equip you with everything you need look and feel great, but knowledge alone is not enough, which brings me to my next point.

You can't do it alone

When left alone, most people become distracted, bored, discouraged and uninspired. If this weren't the case, then there would be hundreds of thousands of people in the 75% group who are happy with how they look and feel. These people don't complete their fitness plans to their full potential or achieve their desired goals because they are trying to achieve them alone: they don't know what to do, and whatever they do know, they're not doing it consistently and so are not committed, and this cycle repeats itself in any of their health and fitness pursuits.

I've met people who have made many mistakes trying to achieve their goals and lost their motivation and confidence in their abilities to look and feel better as a result. What happens? Most people just leave it and don't bother trying again until one of two things happens: inspiration or desperation. They are inspired when they see someone in their social circle with similar challenges who has achieved awesome results and look amazing. The latter is desperation. Most commonly, people act out of desperation when they reach a certain point that is outside of their comfort zone and they need to do something about it before it gets worse. They are feeling older, weaker, unfit, unattractive or frustrated with themselves and their circumstances. They want to come out of this rut so they can feel more energetic, fitter, stronger, look great and feel good about themselves.

Having the right people, professionals and support network will do incredible things for you. In the previous chapters we explored the power of accountability. Do you remember Yvonne in Chapter 2? She is a great example of what it means to have someone there, just like a prime minister has his advisors, or a gymnast has a coach, or a CEO has a mentor. We reach our fullest potential when we're not alone.

Responsibilities, commitments, distractions – repeat

You have children, you work... even if you don't work, looking after children is a full-time job in itself. You might also be a caregiver for a relative or your aging parents. Your annual calendar is booked with work and personal commitments. I know you have responsibilities, commitments and distractions that can get in the way of dedicating time and energy to focus on yourself. I'm not saying it's easy, but it's not impossible either. Everyone has their own set of challenges, but one of life's principles is that things that don't come easy are often the most gratifying when we attain them. That's part of the beauty of achieving a goal, because you've earned it despite your obstacles. Why do you think people get a new sense of confidence, joy and inner power when they achieve the body and mind that they have shaped for themselves? Because they worked hard for it.

The good news is that once you've got the momentum of living a healthier and fitter lifestyle, you just keep going. Many women who've completed their transformation plan have successfully achieved results and maintained them by incorporating it into their lifestyle. They enjoy eating healthier food, they enjoy exercise and miss it when they don't do it, and they feel good for living up to their expectations of how they want to look and feel. It's part of their life.

What to look forward to

Looking and feeling great is the ultimate result. Do you remember we covered your *why* at the start? This is what to look forward to: achieving your why. There is nothing better in life than to be in optimal health and being in a state of good health – by good I mean mentally, physically and emotionally. This creates a beautiful synchronisation. Here is what you can enjoy with good health:

- More energy for day-to-day activities with your kids.

- Healthy, glowing skin that makes you look fresh and vibrant.

- A fuller and more youthful-looking face. (Dehydration and undernourishment can cause the skin to lose its natural vigour and look sunken and sagging.)

- Healthy levels of body fat, so that you can move better. (Body fat impacts your metabolism, blood sugar balance, movement, momentum and emotional wellbeing.)

- Increased self-awareness. Sometimes we get so focused on checking off the items on our to-do list, we forget to check in with ourselves. Focusing on yourself will reduce your stress levels and anxiety and improve your mood and mental state.

- Being able to enjoy food without guilt.

- A healthier gut. What you put into your body is important, but so is what comes out. Having a healthy digestive system will keep your energy levels high, increase your immune system and heighten mental clarity.

- A balanced lifestyle. This is a sign of good health because it means you won't neglect important aspects of your life, such as your loved ones, your fitness and your mental and emotional health.

- Being better able to deal with your own and other people's emotions. When you feel good about yourself it can positively reinforce your thinking.

- Less pain and increased freedom of movement. Joint, bone and muscle health are essential for an active lifestyle, and with regular exercise, you will achieve pain-free motion.

- A stronger immune system to keep you fighting fit and reduce the risk of getting a cold and other illnesses.

To look and feel better, you must embark on your unique fitness journey. The accomplishment of little wins along that journey will build self-confidence. The process of becoming better than you already are is rewarding. You will feel proud of your achievements and gain increased self-respect, which will open the door to self-love. This comes naturally with behavioural change during your fitness journey as you make mindful decisions to better yourself. I've experienced this with clients during their transformation plan – they are more content, not just because of how they look but because they feel good in themselves and that's a great place to be.

Transformation plan success stories

Kathryn

When I first met Kathryn, she had already lost a stone on her own by cutting out anything 'bad' in her diet. Most people take the diet route first when they're on their own because it's the easiest thing to think of and start doing. She had an ambitious but realistic goal of losing four stone within a year. The weight had accumulated over some time, but even more so with her new London lifestyle. At the time Kathryn was a successful recruitment agent and part of her work culture, as in many workplaces in the city, was an end of week drink with colleagues. This, combined with a busy social life with friends and family which involved a lot of eating and drinking, was one of many reasons she found it hard to lose weight and get in shape.

After her initial weight loss Kathryn had hit a plateau and not knowing what to do next, she was referred to me by a colleague. I could tell from our first consultation that she had a 'can do' attitude, which was great recipe for success. Kathryn needed to know what to do, how to do it and when to do it, with support and accountability along the way. Over twelve months and following the 5Ms, Kathryn lost an incredible 21 kg (that's 3 stone and just over three dress sizes). This is a great achievement considering her busy social life. Kathryn didn't miss out on any social events, instead she chose to make healthy choices when she attended them. Her mindset changed and her lifestyle with it. She had a profound respect for her body and was proud of her achievements. Even after we stopped working together, she continued to live a healthier life and joined a netball team to keep up with her exercise. It was certainly a transformational journey for her. We are still friends and keep in contact, and I'm proud to say she has still maintained her results.

Ruth

It was such good fun working with Ruth. We always had a good laugh in the sessions and she had a great energy about her. Ruth is a mum of two lovely children and at the time she was building her new business. Some weight had accumulated after her second pregnancy and she had been stuck at the same size for over two years, so she wanted to get smaller, drop a size and feel better. Food and drink were a barrier and she needed someone to help her keep on top of her diet, so I was excited to introduce her to the daily food accountability challenge. It was a new concept to her, and she felt a little hesitant with my feedback of her daily meals, but she was open to giving it a go.

It worked wonders. Day by day she improved her meals and her portions, she responded well to the feedback and made the effort to stick with it. Combined with exercise sessions, within twelve weeks Ruth lost 7 kg, dropped a dress size and felt really good about herself. She was delighted. When she attended a summer party with many family members and friends, she was showered with compliments. When you haven't seen someone for a while, you can really notice the 'before and after' effect. There were loads of little wins along her fitness journey but that certainly marked a big triumph for Ruth, and she did amazingly well.

Joanne

I was so proud of Joanne's achievements, mainly because she inspired me and showed that age is just a number. Joanne's fitness journey began due to health concerns after she was diagnosed as clinically obese with worryingly high cholesterol. Looking at Joanne, you would never have thought she was obese, but medically, if your body is over a certain range within your age bracket, you're technically within that category. This can create a series of health problems and complications in later life, so Joanne listened to her GP and began to adopt a healthier and more active lifestyle. Her goal was to lose enough weight to fall within the healthy body fat bracket, improve her diet to reduce her cholesterol, and exercise more to get stronger and fitter.

Joanne wasn't a big meat eater, so was surprised by her cholesterol, but her GP said that a variety of foods can cause high cholesterol. She regularly ate pudding after dinner and the butter, cream and other types of fats used in cooking were likely the culprits (along with other factors). To this day I still don't know Joanne's exact age (a gentleman knows better than to ask), but from the hints she gave me, I'd say that she was between her mid-sixties and seventies. After completing her transformation plan, she lost 9 kg (that's nearly a stone and a half) and dropped more than a dress size. More importantly to Joanne, she reduced her cholesterol levels by half – it was the lowest cholesterol level she'd ever had in her life. She was so happy with her results. In her own words, 'I feel really well and energised. I can carry this on forever' – and she did. Joanne continued exercising, which was a big shift in her mindset. I remember her telling me that for her generation, physical exercise wasn't taught. In her youth, exercise and healthy eating wasn't talked about and emphasised, and she didn't grow up in an exercise culture. I'm pleased to say that the habits did stick, and her new healthier way of living became her lifestyle.

Sarah

Sarah had just become a mother when we first met. She had a lovely little boy and although motherhood brought many new experiences and lots of joy, it also had its difficulties. Her goal was to lose her post-baby weight and regain some sort of realistic 'normal' – naturally, the body goes through a lot of changes during pregnancy, and Sarah set herself a realistic view of what to achieve. She needed a fitness routine that was simple, effective and which could easily fit into her life. Although she was busy with her job as a media manager, her baby and planning her wedding, Sarah followed the 5Ms and the results showed. I can happily say she did incredibly well. Sarah lost over 8 kg, she toned up in all the right areas, lost a dress size and fitted perfectly into her stunning wedding dress. I saw her pictures of the big day and she looked amazing – the cut of her dress showed her toned arms, which she loved. Sarah is a testament that no matter what stage of life you're in and whatever you've got going on right now, any time is a good time to focus on yourself. Most of us are busy doing one thing or another, after all, but if you make a choice to work on your mind and body you will look and feel amazing.

Christianne

It's difficult to have any sort of routine in your life when you're constantly travelling, and this was the case for Christianne. She created and managed large corporate events around the world and she loved it because it created many opportunities and experiences, but on the flip side, it took its toll on her body. When I met Christianne her work routine had changed and the opportunity to focus on her health and fitness had presented itself. She was focused on losing the weight, which had crept up over time, and incorporating exercise to feel mentally better and more energised. Laser-focused, we both set out on a mission: she wanted to lose as much healthy weight as possible within the first twelve weeks and I wanted to be sure she did.

You know the 5Ms now. She improved her diet, started to exercise regularly, chose to make positive choices in her lifestyles and took action. The results speak for themselves. I gave Christianne everything she needed but I cannot fault her effort in being consistent. I was impressed at how well she embraced the plan and simply got on with it. In twelve weeks, Christianne lost 15 kg. That's awesome. Her body shape changed; she was slimmer, more toned and more energetic, and she felt great. Everyone works at different paces, and that's fine; it's important to work at your pace for the process to work. Christianne chose to go full steam ahead and it paid off. We had a great time during her journey and she's kept up with this new way of living.

Laura

Laura was an experienced exerciser. She'd done it for many years, but felt she was stuck in a rut and was losing interest. The monotony of her fitness routine was demotivating, and over time she had gained weight. Kickstart was the key theme. Laura needed to kickstart her exercise, diet and mindset to reinvigorate her lifestyle. Her goal was to lose weight and feel better, something she found challenging during the stages of menopause. In her own words, 'I needed to change my mindset.' She didn't go on a diet but welcomed a variety of healthy foods with portions that suited her goals instead of going in and out of strict diets. This made a big difference in helping her to stay motivated and adhere to the transformation plan because she felt she had the freedom to choose what she ate.

Laura lost over 7 kg during the twelve weeks and had more energy than ever before, she felt fantastic. It made a positive impact to her mindset and she felt good about herself. I was so happy when Laura reached her goal because I knew she'd felt frustrated with not seeing any results for a long time. Laura manages a large team and despite the pressures and stress from work combined with raising a child and experiencing changes during menopause, she stuck with it, step by step.

More success stories

We've compiled video case studies of women who have used the five-step method and completed the transformation plan to look and feel great. To see people sharing their stories, visit: www.brigopt.com/success-stories.

Afterword

Congratulations on reading this book and taking steps towards becoming the best version of yourself. I'm glad you have taken the time to focus on you; this is the first step in your fitness journey.

This book has clear themes in it. You have learned the 5Ms – Mindset, Motivation, Meals, Move and Maximise – and how they are all connected to achieve incredible results that can last a lifetime.

You have read other women's experiences and success stories – women who have shown it's possible to look and feel great at any stage in life. You may well have resonated with a particular person and said, 'That's me.'

Feeling good about yourself is vital, and there is no better time than the present to begin your journey to looking and feeling amazing.

Keep it simple and start one step at a time.

Next steps

The BrigoPT transformation plan is a twelve-week program designed for busy, hardworking mothers who want to look great in their clothes, feel confident and lose a dress size or more. The plan is suitable for any woman, whether you're serious about improving your fitness and seeing results or you don't feel that you can commit to a fitness routine on your own and need support on your journey.

To find out more, visit www.brigopt.com.

The Author

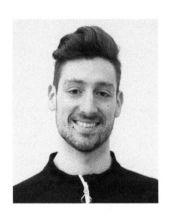

Michael Brigo is a body transformation coach for women with busy lives. He founded Brigo Personal Training in 2015 with the purpose of improving the lives of women who want to look and feel great at any stage in life.

He is recognised as a leading personal trainer for women who has coached hundreds of one-to-one clients with incredible results. He has worked with full-time mothers, business owners, executives and CEOs and coached notable figures such as Nicholas Coleridge, the ex-CEO of Vogue magazine, his wife,

Georgia Coleridge and one of Ford's Super Model of the Year winners, Celia Forner.

BrigoPT's simplistic approach to health, fitness and wellbeing has created an effective way for anyone to lose weight, get in shape and have more energy by providing an all-in-one fitness service in their clients' homes, either in person or by connecting with virtual personal training through their transformation plan.

Contact

🌐 www.brigopt.com

f www.facebook.com/BrigoPT

☉ @brigopt

Lightning Source UK Ltd.
Milton Keynes UK
UKHW051210120921
390336UK00008B/191